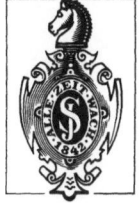

Peter Reeve (Ed.)

Chlamydial Infections

With 20 Figures and 15 Tables

Springer-Verlag Berlin Heidelberg GmbH

Peter Reeve, Ph. D., F. R. C. Path.
Smith Kline & French Laboratories
Research and Development
709 Swedeland Road
Swedeland, PA 19479, USA

ISBN 978-3-540-16552-1   ISBN 978-3-642-71202-9 (eBook)
DOI 10.1007/978-3-642-71202-9

Library of Congress Cataloging in Publication Data
Chlamydial infections. Includes index. 1. Chlamydia infections. I. Reeve, Peter,
1934-[DNLM: 1. Chlamydia Infections. WC 600 C5442] RC124.5.C47 1987 616.9′2
86-26012
ISBN 978-3-540-16552-1

2127/3145-543210

Table of Contents

List of Contributors

Bowie, William R., M. D., F. R. C. P. (C)
Division of Infectious Diseases, University of British Columbia,
910 W. 10th Avenue, Vancouver B. C. V5Z 1M9, Canada

Byrne, Gerald I., M. D.
Department of Medical Microbiology,
University of Wisconsin-Madison,
Medical School, Madison, WI 53706, USA

Hammerschlag, Margaret R., M. D.
Department of Pediatrics, Downstate Medical Center,
450 Clarkson Avenue, Brooklyn, N. Y. 11203, USA

Hanna, Lavelle, Ph. D.
Department of Microbiology, S-412, University of California,
San Francisco, San Francisco, CA 94143, USA

Hipp, Sally Sloan, Ph. D.
STD Laboratory, Wadsworth Center for Laboratories and Research,
New York State Department of Health, Albany, N. Y. 12201, USA

Keat, Andrew C. S., M. D., M. R. C. P.
St. Stephen's Hospital, Fulham Road, Chelsea SW10 9TH,
Great Britain

Mårdh, Per-Anders, M. D.
Institute of Clinical Bacteriology, University of Uppsala,
Box 552, 751 22 Uppsala, Sweden

Reeve, Peter, Ph. D., F. R. C. Path.
Smith Kline & French Laboratories, Research and Development,
709 Swedeland Road, Swedeland, PA 19479, USA.

Schachter, Julius, Ph. D.
Chlamydia Laboratory, Department of Laboratory Medicine,
San Francisco General Hospital, Building 30, Room 416,
San Francisco, CA 94110, USA

Stamm, Walter E., M. D.
Division of Infectious Diseases, Department of Medicine,
Harborview Medical Center, 325 Ninth Avenue, Seattle,
WA 98104, USA

Introduction

Peter Reeve[1] and Lavelle Hanna[2]

[1]Smith Kline & French Laboratories, Research and Development, 709 Swedeland Road, Swedeland, PA 19479, USA
[2]Department of Microbiology, S-412, University of California, San Francisco, San Francisco, CA 94143, USA

Trachoma, an infectious keratoconjunctivitis due to chlamydial infection, was one of the earliest recognized clinical entities. References to it have been noted in Egyptian papyri and in Greco-Roman medical treatises. Since those times it has remained a most important eye infection, and indeed trachoma is still a major cause of blindness in rural communities, affecting probably 6 million people (Dawson).

The causal agent of trachoma was identified by Halberstaeter and von Provazek in a much-quoted but little-read paper published over 75 years ago. It was after the isolation and demonstration of the growth of the causal agent of trachoma, *Chlamydia trachomatis,* by Tang and his colleagues in China in the late 1950s that there was an enormous increase in our knowledge of these agents. The real explosion of knowledge and interest in *Chlamydia,* however, has been in the last decade. With the growing awareness of the extraordinary commonness of chlamydial infections, not only in developing countries but also in the highly developed countries, has come a considerable interest from all areas concerned with medical science, from clinicians to molecular biologists.

It is now clear that *Chlamydia* is one of the most prevalent of infectious organisms and causal relationships are now known to exist between *Chlamydia* and eye infections, genital infections, and infections of the newborn; *Chlamydia* can cause acute and chronic infections and evidence of this group is now sought wherever there are disorders of unknown or obscure etiology.

Early in this century, association of *Chlamydia* with many veterinary infections and with human genital tract disease was observed, but interest in the infections remained limited to veterinarians, ophthalmologists, microbiologists, and pathologists. As a result, most students attending medical school before 1970 completed their microbiology and infectious disease training without having heard even the word *"Chlamydia."*

The genus *Chlamydia* is a bacterium which is an obligatory intracellular parasite, dependent upon the host cell for its energy. There are currently two species described: *C. trachomatis,* which is associated with human disease, and *C. psittaci,* which is associated with animal diseases and rarely transferred to a human host. The chapter Biology of the Chlamydiae provides a general description of the agent.

In 1895 Morange applied the name "psittacosis" to a disease of psittacine birds, which was sometimes transmitted to human contacts in the form of a pneumonia. In 1912 another entity was recognized which is now known as lymphogranuloma

Chlamydial Infections
Edited by P. Reeve
© Springer-Verlag Berlin Heidelberg 1987

venereum (LGV). Proof of etiology was slow, but in the 1930s chlamydiae were isolated in mice and in chick embryos infected with both psittacosis and LGV.

The first laboratory evidence of an infective agent of trachoma was the demonstration by Halberstaeter and Provazek in 1907 that scrapings from a trachomatous eye could produce subclinical to mild conjunctivitis in orangutans, and that cytologic examination of conjunctival scrapings from both natural and experimental hosts revealed the presence of "inclusion bodies" (really a micro colony of bacteria within cellular cytoplasm) with varying morphology. During the next few years, Lindner and Halberstaeter and Provazek described similar inclusions in conjunctival scrapings from infants with nongonococcal ophthalmia neonatorum and in cervical and urethral specimens from their parents.

Sequential microscopic studies of experimentally infected subjects showed a characteristic pattern of development regardless of the clinical disease from which the infectious agent came, with an infectious "elementary body" entering a susceptible cell, reorganizing to a larger, less dense, noninfectious "initial body" (now referred to as a "reticulum body"), and completing the cycle with release of the infectious elementary body.

The report by Tang et al. describing isolation of the trachoma agent in chick embryo yolk sac was soon confirmed by Collier and Sowa in the Gambia, and was followed by isolations in the United States, Saudi Arabia, Israel and Taiwan. Isolation of *C. trachomatis* from neonates with inclusion conjunctivitis and from their mothers by Jones et al. was soon confirmed by Hanna et al. But isolation in chick embryo yolk sac remained a cumbersome, slow procedure. In 1965 Gordon and Quan described isolations in irradiated cultured cells following centrifugation of the inoculum onto monolayers. It is now recognized that the centrifugation was the important step in the procedure and to date it is essential. Modifications reported in the basic procedure reflect those of individual laboratories.

According to World Health Organization (WHO) figures, four to five hundred million people (more than one-tenth of the population of the world) have trachoma. No adequate information is available for genital infection, but following the rapidly increasing rate of infection with all sexually transmissible diseases, this has become a major problem. Nongonococcal urethritis and cervicitis are not reportable diseases in the United States, but in Western Europe and the United Kingdom chlamydial infection appears to be far more frequent than gonorrhea.

Until 1938, treatment of trachoma had not progressed from Egyptian times, and consisted of vigorous scraping of the conjunctiva, surgery, or scraping with "blue stone," i. e., copper sulfate - all more traumatic and painful than the affliction itself. The availability of sulfanilamide changed therapeutic practices, and this drug appeared to cure the infection. However, it did not eradicate the chlamydiae from populations, and was later replaced by the tetracyclines as drug of choice.

During the past 20 years there have been many volumes published on the subject. However, most of these have been directed toward research workers. The chapters of this volume have been assembled in the hope of gathering together information pertinent to the clinician. We hope to alert general practitioners, internists, pediatricians, gynecologists, urologists, and public health personnel - in addition to microbiologists and ophthalmologists - to the importance of chlamydial infections and to provide some practical guidance in laboratory diagnostic methods and treatment. Since 1907 much progress has been made in understanding chlamydial infections, but our information is far from adequate. We have practical methods of isolating the agent, but these appear to be insensitive. Other, unrecognized agents may be responsible for the unexplained nongonococcal urethritis and cervicitis, but the prevalence of chlamydial antibodies in the general population does not support this. As isolation techniques improve and as serological procedures become increasingly sensitive, we can hope for further knowledge.

Until recently, the latest techniques of modern biotechnology, using recon DNA and molecular genetics, monoclonal antibodies and peptide synthesis, had not been applied intensively to the study of *Chlamydia*. Lately, the use of monoclonal antibodies has provided rapid diagnostic techniques and it may be that definitive microbiological diagnosis of *Chlamydia* infections will possibly be accomplished in a few minutes in a doctor's practice or clinic, and the specialized and expensive laboratory procedures currently used will no longer be necessary.

What will we do with all this knowledge? Much remains to be done, even now, on the epidemiology of chlamydial infections. There are unanswered questions about the association of infections by *C. trachomatis* of such remote anatomical sites as the eye and genital tract with geographic location and socioeconomic class. Why is trachoma predominantly an eye infection of developing and especially arid countries, while genital infections (and associated diseases of the newborn) occur predominantly in the large urban areas of developed countries? Is there a genital infection with trachoma, unnoticed because as yet unsought or undemonstrated? What is the biological and molecular basis for the apparent extraordinary tissue specificity of ocular and genital biovars?

If etiology and epidemiology are assured of continued study, and more is learned of the biology of these agents as recom DNA and other techniques are applied, what can we expect of control and treatment? In spite of the prevalence of chlamydial infections and the inconvenience, pain, suffering, and economic loss which they cause, there are virtually no studies directed solely at control of infection by seeking specific antichlamydial drugs or treatments. Recently, the Sandoz Research Institute in Vienna has specifically sought to demonstrate antichlamydial activity of new synthetic drugs. Further studies are reported on rifampicin derivatives developed specifically for antichlamydial treatment. In all other cases the existing drugs are for specific antichlamydial treatment screened by in vitro test procedures or evaluated in clinical trials or still use antibiotics such as the tetracyclines and erythromycins which have been known for 20 years. New studies concern the subtleties of treatment schedules rather than testing new drugs.

If the search for truly antichlamydial drugs has proved so unattractive, what about immunological control? Why not control by vaccination? Many studies done in the 1960s by several large research groups in the United States, United Kingdom, and Saudi Arabia had as their goal the control of trachoma by vaccination. Unfortunately, in spite of some limited success in inducing short-term immunity in baboons, there was no indication at all that vaccination will prove successful. The superficiality of infection, the poor immunological stimulation, and the lack of access for the circulating antibody to the infecting organism seem to militate against the prospects of chlamydial vaccines. Again, there are a large number of chlamydial serovars and the significance of these for immunity is unknown.

A complex laboratory classification has been built up on detailed serological cross-reactions between chlamydial serovars. How significant these are in medical terms and how far they represent minute gradings of merely laboratory significance is a question that needs resolution. New immunological and biological diagnostic techniques would help to resolve it.

With the advent of new rapid diagnostic techniques and the application of the methods of molecular genetics and immunology, we can anticipate a new expansion of our knowledge and a concomitant increase in the literature, with not only the devotion of more space to the subject in relevant scientific journals but perhaps even specific journals concerned solely with *Chlamydia*.

To paraphrase Nocard, who stated, *"La psittacose n'existe pas, si elle existe, elle est partout,"* chlamydiae exist, and they are everywhere.

Laboratory Diagnosis of Chlamydial Infection

Sally Sloan Hipp

STD Laboratory, Wadsworth Center for Laboratories and Research, New York. State Department of Health, Albany, N.Y. 12201, USA

Laboratory Identification of *Chlamydia trachomatis*

No single test for laboratory identification of chlamydial infection is entirely satisfactory. Three approaches have commonly been used: visualization of inclusions in direct smears, serologic methods, and growth of the organism from clinical specimens in tissue culture. All three methods have specific areas of usefulness, as well as drawbacks which limit their applicability.

Tissue culture, although a tedious and imperfect system, is nonetheless the most sensitive and reliable way to incriminate *Chlamydia* as being associated with present infections. Therefore, the cytologic and serologic approaches will be summarized briefly and the culture procedure described in more detail.

Recently, two commercial rapid diagnostic tests have become available, and although these are presently being evaluated for usefulness, some information is available as to their potential applicability in the laboratory.

Cytology

Cytologic staining of chlamydial inclusions is most useful in cases of eye infection, where inclusions are numerous and the samples are relatively free of debris which may obscure the inclusions. For direct genital scrapings, where the converse is true, the usefulness of this approach is limited. Great care must be exercised when attempting cytologic identification of *Chlamydia* from sites other than the eye. Artifacts are common and inclusions do not always look typical. Giemsa and fluorescent antibody staining of inclusions are the most common of these cytologic procedures [20, 63]. Papanicolaou stain is also used to identify genital chlamydial inclusions [18], but confirmation by cell culture is strongly recommended [25], and in a recent comparative study of cytology with cultural identification of *Chlamydia*, Shafer et al. [67] concluded that cytology is not useful as a definitive method for diagnosis of chlamydial infection.

Chlamydial Infections
Edited by P. Reeve
© Springer-Verlag Berlin Heidelberg 1987

Serology

Serologic tests for chlamydial infection are rapidly evolving [77], and as the immunology of *Chlamydia* [38] becomes better understood and monoclonal antibodies [71] become available for definition of antigen specificities, serology may eventually emerge as the test of choice. This approach is convenient because samples are easily obtained, results are available more rapidly than by culture, and there are no fragile organisms to be kept alive during transport to the laboratory. The basic limitation at present to serologic diagnosis of chlamydial infection is that a high background of chlamydial antibodies in some populations [65] makes it difficult to relate titers to present infections in individual cases. Several broad types of serologic tests are used to detect or confirm *Chlamydia* infections:

Complement Fixation

The complement fixation (CF) test is widely familiar – it was used for diagnosis of lymphogranuloma venereum (LGV; see section with this title below) and psittacosis long before the prevalence of genital chlamydial infections became known – and so it is widely but inappropriately used for confirmatory chlamydial serology. This test is based on a genus-specific antigen which recognizes all *Chlamydia* organisms, but because high titers to this antigen do not develop following adult ocular or genital infections, the test is practically useless for current, common *Chlamydia* infections. This irrelevance, however, is neither clearly understood by many who request the test nor clearly stated by those who provide it.

Microimmunofluorescence

The microimmunofluorescence (MIF) test [80], which employs as antigen a combination of all 14 strains of *Chlamydia trachomatis,* has the advantage of being both specific and sensitive. The test is performed by placing solutions of all 14 antigens in microdot clusters on a microscope slide; after these are dried, dilutions of patient sera followed by fluorescein-labeled antihuman antibodies are added. The microdots are then examined for specific fluorescence. The 14 antigens can be replaced by four antigen pools representing genital, trachoma, LGV, and psittacosis serotypes [78]. The antihuman fluorescein conjugate can comprise antisera reacting with IgM, IgA, or IgG, thus permitting the detection of specific classes of antibodies. Such modifications permit the introduction of both versatility and simplification into this test. A detailed step-by-step procedure for MIF has been prepared by Bird et al. [5]. Few laboratories, however, are equipped for the extensive procedures necessary to prepare the antigen. The test is therefore not yet widely available for routine testing.

A recent study by Schachter et al. [66] of infants with pneumonia has indicated that MIF may be the diagnostic method of choice in such cases. Cultural identification of *Chlamydia* did not appear to be as reliable or as sensitive as IgM antibodies for indicating infection. Also, results with MIF can be obtained the same day, while culture takes 2 or 3 days. Such studies indicating a specific usefulness for MIF may well have a positive influence on its future availability.

Enzyme-Linked Immunosorbent Assay

The enzyme-linked immunosorbent assay (ELISA) has gained widespread acceptance in diagnostic microbiology because it is easy to perform and can readily be adapted to a wide variety of infections. In a few studies evaluating this test for detection of chlamydial antibodies [9, 42, 43], the ELISA method has been shown to be more sensitive, more specific, and less expensive to perform than CF or MIF but subject to the same limits as the other serologic methods for detection of present chlamydial infection. A recent study [16] indicates that this method is more sensitive for detection of IgG than of IgM antibodies.

Single-Antigen Indirect Fluorescence

The single-antigen indirect fluorescence (IF) test, as developed by Richmond and Caul [57] and Saikku and Paavonen [61], employs whole chlamydial inclusions for a single serotype as antigen. This test is easy to initiate when cell culture facilities are available. In our experience this test is simple, inexpensive, and convenient to perform; using the L2 serotypes it has proved to be a useful supplement to the culture program in this laboratory.

Increased public awareness of chlamydial disease has led to increased demands for methods for detecting this organism. A serologic test specific for present chlamydial infection would be extremely valuable, especially for women. Since many women would prefer to have a blood sample rather that a cervical sample taken, and since most women with chlamydial infection have no signs or symptoms indicative of this disease, serology could identify cases that might otherwise be missed. Serology is also particularly useful in identifying cases where *Chlamydia* cannot always be isolated with great reliability, as in infant pneumonia or adult proctitis. Although commercial tests are rapidly becoming available, their usefulness awaits confirmatory, independent evaluation. One recent evaluation of a commercial IF test reflects the dilemma inherent in the development of serologic diagnosis. In this study [35] the IF test was positive for 28 of 30 culture-positive specimens, while 142 of 169 culture-negative patients (with presumptive chlamydial infection) were also IF positive. These results may indicate low sensitivity of culture or false-positive results by serology. Until more studies and confirmatory evaluations become available, serologic testing for chlamydial infection will probably continue to find greatest usefulness in epidemiologic studies.

Tissue Culture

The significance of *Chlamydia* as a sexually transmissible agent has been recognized only recently, and appropriate methodology for specimen handling from collection through culture is still evolving. Optimum sensitivity is achieved only when appropriate specimens are properly collected, properly transported, and cultured under stringently controlled procedures. Such results require cooperation and good communication between clinicians and the laboratory.

Specimens

The low isolation rate often encountered by laboratory workers just beginning chlamydial cultures may be due to low incidence in the population being tested, but more probably the samples may not have been taken from appropriate body sites. Samples from which *Chlamydia* can routinely be isolated successfully are listed in Table 1.

Because *C. trachomatis* inhabits columnar epithelial cells of the genital tract, samples taken for culture must contain these cells. The most appropriate samples from women are cells from both the endocervix and urethra [30, 53]. For samples from men urethral discharge is not adequate; the samples should be obtained by inserting a swab 2–5 cm into the urethra and rotating it gently to obtain cellular material. However, seminal fluid [21] and several of its components [51] may interfere with the ability of *C. trachomatis* to form inclusions in cell culture.

Laparoscopic samples from the fallopian tubes have yielded *C. trachomatis* in cases of salpingitis [49] and in infertile woman with tubal obstruction [24]. Routine culture for *Mycoplasma* and *Ureaplasma* should be included in laparoscopic evaluations, since these organisms have also been isolated from patients with infertility [23] and salpingitis [47]; neither organism will be found unless specific tests are included. In most hospitals in the United States laparoscopy is not routinely performed in cases of pelvic inflammatory disease, so the possible involvement of *C. trachomatis* must often be inferred from isolation of this organism from the cervices of patients with symptoms.

For infants with suspected chlamydial infection, conjunctival swabs and nasopharyngeal aspirates can be tested. In this laboratory we request that both specimens be sent, even though no eye symptoms may be present. When *Chlamydia* is present, it is easy to isolate from babies' eyes, and positive cultures have been obtained from infants with only pneumonia-like symptoms, even when nasopharyngeal aspirates were negative.

In our experience the most unrewarding populations for chlamydial isolation

Table 1. Appropriate samples for culture of *Chlamydia*

Source	Specimen	Comments
Male genital		
Urethra	Swab	Insert swab 2–5 cm, rotate firmly to obtain cellular material; discharge is unsatisfactory.
Epididymis	Aspirate	
Female genital	Cells from	Sample both urethra and cervix for
Cervix	cervical os	improved isolation; discharge is not satisfactory.
Fallopian tubes	Biopsy material	Test for *Ureaplasma* also.
Eye	Swab of lower conjunctiva	
Rectum	Swab of anorectal mucous membrane	Bacterial contamination from feces often overgrows culture.
Nasopharynx (Infant with pneumonia)	Nasopharyngeal aspirate	Send conjunctival swab also; *Chlamydia* is sometimes isolated from asymptomatic eyes.

have been cervical specimens sent from vaginitis patients [19] or infertility patients [79], yet requests for such tests are common. Routine testing of samples such as urine sediment and urine [3, 69] or vaginal discharge is a waste of time and effort and should be discouraged by the laboratory. Attempts to isolate the organism from men with prostatitis have also been unsuccessful [50], although female partners of such patients may sometimes yield positive cultures [76]. Partner testing may be useful in cases of female genital infection as well. Female genital samples often contain either heavy bacterial contamination or substances toxic to cells, making it impossible to determine whether *Chlamydia* is present. In these cases testing urethral samples from a regular consort may provide presumptive confirmation.

Various vaginal preparations, including douches, spermicides, and diaphragm creams, may either inhibit the growth of *Chlamydia* [52] or cause toxicity in cell cultures [28]. Therefore, negative cultures of specimens from women who have used these preparations within 24 h of testing may be invalid.

Transport of Specimens

As the time of transport from clinic to laboratory increases, the isolation rate of *Chlamydia* from clinical specimens tends to decline. This problem does not often arise in England or Scandinavia, where clinics and laboratories are frequently in close proximity. Since much of the early developmental work on genital chlamydial cultures has come from those countries, there is a paucity of information on transport systems. In the United States, however, the specimens must often be shipped some distance for testing, and this can be a factor in a failure to recover *Chlamydia*.

Most specimens for transport are placed in 2SP transport medium, which contains added 3% fetal bovine serum (FBS) [11] and antibiotics; a sorbitol buffer [56] is also useful to maintain viability of *Chlamydia* during transport. We have found that survival of *Chlamydia* is improved by a mixture of equal parts 2SP and growth medium, but this must be used within 2 weeks of preparation; 2SP alone can be stored frozen for about 3 months before use. Wooden stick swabs are inhibitory to *Chlamydia* [48] and must never be left in the transport medium. Samples to be transported within 24 h should be kept cold but not frozen. For longer delays freezing and storage at $-70\,°C$ is necessary; this requires the use of Dry Ice for transport and raises the shipping cost considerably.

There is a great need for a transport system that can maintain the viability of *C. trachomatis* for at least 48 h at room temperature. With the advent of centralized commercial culture testing services for this organism the necessity becomes even more apparent. Specimens should not be stored at $-20\,°C$. The extreme loss of viability after 24 h of $-20\,°C$ storage is shown in Table 2 and has been previously noted by others [13].

An interesting approach by Ridgeway et al. [58] suggests a method that might overcome the problem of specimen transport. Their reference laboratory provided coverslip cell cultures for the local laboratory, which were then inoculated, incubated, and interpreted on site. With replicate specimens, results obtained on site were slightly better than were those obtained by the reference laboratory, with 12 of 58 positives obtained only at the local laboratory. Prepared cell cultures were sent to the local laboratory twice a week. Such a method can obviate costly and undesirable

Table 2. Effects of storage temperature upon recovery of *C. trachomatis*[a]

Storage temperature (°C)	Average no. of inclusions/coverslip		
	Original suspension	After 24 h storage	Recovery (%)
5	322	210	65
−20	286	68	23
−70	232	292	100+
−20/−70[b]	288	8	3

[a] A laboratory strain of *C. trachomatis* (male urethral isolate) was used in this experiment. The organism was prepared for testing by disrupting an infected culture by using a vibrating mixer and filtering the fluid through a 0.8-μm filter. The filtrate was diluted 1:10 into 2SP transport medium, and an estimate of the original concentrations of *Chlamydia* was obtained by immediate inoculation into 2-day McCoy cell monolayers treated with cytochalasin B. Each sample was then stored at the indicated temperature for 24 h, thawed rapidly in tepid water, and retested. Each count is the average of duplicate cover slips.
[b] This sample was frozen and held at −20 °C for 24 h, moved to −70 °C for another 24 h, and then thawed and retested.

transport as well as ensuring uniform quality of the tissue culture cells. A major challenge of *Chlamydia* isolation is the quality control necessary to assure that tissue culture cells will support the growth of this organism in a sensitive and reproducible manner. Personnel of clinics with laboratory facilities can easily be trained to carry out the inoculation and staining procedures and even the examination of the stained smears. This method may be the optimal way for reference laboratories to get other laboratories started in chlamydial culture programs.

Although several commercial companies now sell prepared cell tubes which can be inoculated and processed by the clinics, it is well initially to carry out a comparative evaluation of these. We have found that some of the cells are often quite old, and thus quite dense when inoculated. This can obscure the reading of inclusions.

Cell Culture Techniques

Inoculation of tissue cultures, most commonly of McCoy cells [17], is used for isolation of *C. trachomatis*. If the organism is present, after incubation intracytoplasmic inclusions will readily be visualized microscopically by iodine, Giemsa, or fluorescent antibody staining. Results of testing are generally available 2–3 days after the specimens are inoculated into cell culture, although one report [75] indicates that it is possible to achieve results in less than 24 h by using a combination of cycloheximide-treated cells and immunofluorescence staining.

The development of tissue culture techniques for *Chlamydia* has been well documented by Hobson [29]. In addition to McCoy cells (mouse L cells) several other tissue culture cell lines can be used to grow *Chlamydia*, including BHK-21 [44] and Hela 229 [10]. As a rule these are used by the groups that developed them. McCoy cells seem now to have the broadest usage and are available commercially from M.A. Bioproducts (Walkersville, Maryland) or can often be obtained as a gift from a virus or *Chlamydia* laboratory. Those from the latter, however, frequently contain *Mycoplasma* contamination, whereas the commercial cells are guaranteed *Mycoplasma*-free.

Pretreatment of the cells is necessary for optimal growth of *Chlamydia*. A variety of suitable pretreatment methods are used, including irradiation [17] or incubation with diethylaminoethyl dextran [37], cycloheximide [59], 5-iodo-2'-deoxyuridine [82], or cytochalasin B [70].

Our laboratory has used cytochalasin B because the large, bright inclusions that are formed in such cultures make identification rapid and simple. Reports [15, 40], while noting these qualities, found that cycloheximide gave many more inclusions, although of lesser size and brightness. As a result of these reports we now use a combination of both chemicals – a modification of the method of Sompolinsky and Richmond [70] according to which cells are grown in cytochalasin B and cycloheximide is added after specimen inoculation. This technique gives both high numbers and high quality of inclusions, while having no detrimental effects upon the isolation (S.S. Hipp, unpublished observation), and seems ideal for workers with no experience who are just beginning a *Chlamydia* identification system.

McCoy cells are grown and maintained in flasks in Eagle minimal essential medium, supplemented with Earl's balanced salt solution plus 10% (vol/vol) FBS and

Table 3. Materials used for *Chlamydia* isolation with McCoy cells treated with cytochalasin B and cycloheximide

Growth medium	Eagle minimal essential	
	Earl's Powder (Gibco, Grand Island, New York)	9.52 g
	NaHCO$_3$	2.2 g
	Phenol red (1% solution)	2.0 ml
	Streptomycin sulfate	0.05 g
	Nystatin	25 000 units
	Vancomycin	100 mg
	Millipore H$_2$O to make 1 l	
	Add FBS	100 ml
McCoy cells	Add 10% (vol/vol) dimethyl sulfoxide (DMSO) to multiple samples (1 ml each) of newly purchased cell suspensions. Store in 1-ml amounts in liquid N$_2$. To start a new cell line, thaw a vial quickly at 37 °C, pipette contents into tissue culture flask containing 20 ml growth medium, incubate flask at 37 °C overnight, and change the medium to remove DMSO. Cells in each flask are passaged when confluent (4–5 days). Discard after 25 passages.	
Trypsin-Versene [45]	NaCl	8.0 g
	KCL	0.4 g
	Dextrose	1.0 g
	NaHCO$_3$	0.58 g
	Disodium EDTA (ethylenediaminetetraacetic acid)	
		0.2 g
	Millipore H$_2$O	1000 ml
	Trypsin	0.5 g
	Sterile filter	
2 SP transport medium [83]	Sucrose	68.46 g

Table 3. (continued)

	Anhydrous K_2HPO_4	2.008 g
	Anhydrous KH_2PO_4	1.088 g
	Millipore H_2O	1000 ml
	FBS	30 ml
	Antibiotics	As for growth medium
	This can be stored frozen for 3 months; for better survival of organisms during transport mix 1:1 with growth medium before inoculation.	
Cytochalasin B	Weigh out cyt B powder (handle with extreme care) and dissolve in DMSO at 1 mg/ml. Dispense solution in 0.1-ml amounts into small vials and freeze in liquid N_2. For working solution add 0.9 ml growth medium to vial.	
Cycloheximide	Weigh out as for cyt B and dissolve powder in H_2O. Store as for cyt B. Add to inoculated cell tubes 1 h after centrifugation.	
Stains		
Giemsa	Giemsa concentrate (Fisher Scientific, Fairlawn, New Jersey)	2 ml
	$1/15\,M$ sodium phosphate buffer	50 ml
Iodine	KI	5 g
	Iodine crystals	5 g
	95% ethanol	50 ml
	H_2O	50 ml
NaCl	Cell cultures are stained in Nunc tubes. Remove medium, rinse with phosphate-buffered NaCl, fix cells with 1 ml methanol for 10 min. Remove MeOH. Rinse with phosphate buffer and stain with either I (2 min) or Giemsa (30 min). After staining remove coverslip by poking hot needle through bottom of tube. Mounting fluid I stain: I to glycerol (1:3). Mounting fluid Giemsa: Permount (Fisher Scientific, Fairlawn, New Jersey).	

0.2% $NaHCO_3$ (Table 3). To prepare monolayers the cells are removed from the flasks with trypsin-Versene and diluted to 1×10^5 cells/ml with growth medium containing 2 µg cytochalasin B per milliliter. This suspension is dispensed in 1-ml amounts into flat-bottomed, plastic Nunc tubes (Vanguard, Neptune, New Jersey), each containing a 10-mm-diameter coverslip (Rochester Scientific, Rochester, New York). The tubes are incubated for 2 days at 35 °C to form a confluent cell layer. One tube is stained prior to inoculation to ensure that the cells have grown well. The monolayer tubes are inoculated in triplicate with clinical specimens, centrifuged at $2000 \times g$ for 1 h at 30°–35 °C, and incubated for at least 1 h [31]. Then the medium is changed to a fresh growth medium which contains 1 µg cytochalasin B and 1 µg cycloheximide per milliliter plus antibiotics. The inoculated tubes are incubated for 2 days, after which time one tube is stained with iodine or fluorescent antibody; the following day a second tube is stained with Giemsa. The third tube is either discarded or passaged to increase the number of inclusions, as necessary.

Many laboratories use only iodine staining for chlamydial identification because the results are available 1 day earlier than with Giemsa and the staining procedure is more rapid. However, care must be taken when using iodine stain to avoid false-positive results due to a variety of artifacts, including glycogen-containing epithelial cells found in some female genital specimens; talcum powder from the physician's examining gloves may also look like iodine-stained inclusions [26]. Bright-field observation may be used in conjunction with Giemsa staining to detect inclusions, but this method requires much experience for accurate reading of samples with low inclusion counts, as cell vacuoles sometimes look like inclusions. Dark-field viewing of the same Giemsa-stained slides, however, provides a remarkably distinct identification of *Chlamydia;* the inclusions appear bright, autofluorescent green against a background of McCoy cells with brown cytoplasm and purple-blue nuclei. This technique is particularly useful with cycloheximide-treated cells, where iodine-stained inclusions are sometimes small, lightly stained, and difficult for the inexperienced to discern. This laboratory has recently tested over 300 clinical specimens using all three methods of staining – iodine, Giemsa, and commercial monoclonal fluorescent antibody (FA) (Bartels Immunodiagnostics, Seattle, Washington). Of these specimens, 24 were culture positive for *Chlamydia* by one or more staining techniques. In eight of these the Giemsa was negative, as was the iodine in four specimens. The FA was always positive and in most cases gave much higher inclusion counts than either of the other stains.

A recent study by Hipp et al. [27] found that McCoy cell suspensions could conveniently be substituted for preformed monolayers for inoculation with *Chlamydia*. The use of cell suspensions eliminates the necessity of estimating the number of specimens to be processed on future days, since suspensions can be inoculated immediately upon preparation. It was further noted that monolayers of from 1 to 4 days of age were all satisfactory for recovery of *Chlamydia*. Monolayers older than 4 days tended to have heavy growth that sometimes obscured the inclusions; use of these older cultures is therefore not recommended.

Quality Control
Several aspects of quality control are essential to successful tissue culture isolation of *C. trachomatis*.

Assay Variables. Periodically, the culture system may cease to function well for reasons which are not readily apparent. A variety of factors can affect the growth of *C. trachomatis*, including temperature, the pH of the medium, the CO_2 concentration [31], the glass- or plasticware used [68], the collection tubes and swabs [48], exposure of the organism to penicillin [32], and toxicity of some lots of cycloheximide [7]. If careful records are kept – e.g., lots of trypsin and numbers of medium constituents, changes of temperature, and passage numbers – it may be possible to trace the source of the problem; however, the best solution often is to discard all the cultures and start over again with fresh cells, positive controls, and medium.

Chlamydia must be centrifuged onto the cell monolayer in order to achieve optimal uptake and growth in the cell culture. The speed, duration, and temperature of centrifugation are all important. Johnson and Hobson [31] showed that an uncentrifuged sample yielded 60 inclusions, while the same sample centrifuged at $2500 \times g$ or $4500 \times g$ for 1 h gave 3100 and 23 400 inclusions respectively. Darougar et al. [12] determined that centrifugation at 35 °C would give four times the numbers of inclusions obtained at ambient temperature. Elevation of centrifugation temperature can often be achieved naturally in old centrifuges simply from the heat of the motor. Such runs should be monitored frequently by measuring the final temperature of uninoculated cells.

Controls. A positive control culture of *C. trachomatis* must be passaged along continually with the culture system to ensure that the organism can indeed be isolated. Strains of LGV do not make suitable control cultures; they will grow profusely under conditions that do not support the growth of other chlamydial strains and will thus give a distorted picture of the sensitivity of the system. Because LGV grows so well, specimens or even cell cultures can easily be contaminated with this organism; it should not be grown near a routine isolation system.

Almost any chlamydial strain, if passaged often enough, will adapt to tissue culture and grow better than isolates from clinical specimens. Therefore, additional sensitivity checks can be obtained by use of a population control. This entails performing routine culture for high-risk-group patients, such as persons with gonorrhea, those with nonspecific urethritis and their consorts, or men with postgonococcal urethritis. Such groups would be expected to yield isolates in one of every three or four specimens [54]. If numbers approaching this prevalence are not found, the isolation system may need reevaluation.

Fetal Bovine Serum. Screening of each lot of FBS used in the medium is critical to isolation of *C. trachomatis.* Some lots will grow tissue culture cells but suppress inclusion formation [14]. Newborn calf serum should not be substituted for FBS [39].

Rapid Diagnostic Tests

Recently, two commercial tests have been developed which seem to offer alternatives to tissue culture for detection of chlamydial infection. These are MicroTrak, a direct monoclonal antibody test (Syva Company, Palo Alto, California), and Chlamydiazyme, an enzyme-linked immunoassay (Abbott Labs., Chicago, Illinois). Although both of these tests have received wide publicity heralding their potential, there is so far little comparative independent scientific evaluation of their performance available.

The MicroTrak test employs a fluorescein-conjugated monoclonal antibody to *C. trachomatis* which is used to identify elementary particles in a direct smear. A sample from a urogenital swab is placed on a slide and fixed by the clinician, then sent to a laboratory for fluorescent staining and inspection. The potential advantages of this test are immediate results (30 min versus 3 days for cell culture), no requirement for elaborate Dry Ice transport, and reduced cost (about $ 6 for materials only).

The initial evaluation of MicroTrak by the group involved in the development of the test [72] found it to be 93% sensitive and 96% specific when applied to a symptomatic population with high incidence of sexually transmissible disease. Similar results were obtained by Quinn et al. [55] in both symptomatic and asymptomatic populations with high prevalence rates. Beyond this, independent data are just now becoming available. Several letters to editors have appeared making brief comments on MicroTrak, two of which [46, 60] found culture performed better, while two others [4, 22] indicated the direct test to have advantages over culture. One other letter [73] reported the successful preliminary use of MicroTrak for identifying *C. trachomatis* in eye infections. A recent report [36] has pointed out that MicroTrak reagent stains staphylococci due to the binding of protein A, thus giving rise to the possibility of false-positive readings by inexperienced workers. The likelihood of false-positives has also been pointed out by others [74].

From the work so far in our laboratory, several practical observations can be made regarding testing procedures. The fluorescent-stained elementary particles are very small even at × 100 magnification, and other materials of generally the same size and color can be seen in smears. Thus it is imperative that an excellent-quality fluorescent microscope with perfect alignment be used. It is also necessary to have some training to discern positive from negative specimens; such training would best be obtained from a Syva representative. Although the ultimate usefulness of this test awaits evaluation by competently trained investigators, it seems likely that it will provide some useful supplement to cell culture. It further seems likely that it will be found most useful in those samples that are easiest to identify in cell culture due to their large numbers of inclusions and relative lack of interfering substances, i.e., conjunctival swabs and male urethral specimens.

Little information has so far appeared regarding Chlamydiazyme. The basis of this test is that any chlamydial antigen contained in a urogenital sample will be absorbed to a polystyrene bead, coupled to *C. trachomatis* antibody, and then detected colorimetrically after reaction with horseradish-peroxidase-conjugated antibody and chromogen. The potential advantages are the same as for MicroTrak: decreased testing time (4 h), decreased cost, and simplified transport.

Three abstracts of presentations [2, 33, 41] indicated general agreement of Chlamydiazyme results with cell culture, although there was some observation of low sensitivity (75%). Two full papers [1, 34], one an extension of one of these abstracts, have so far evaluated Chlamydiazyme. However, since the work was done for these studies the company has reworked the test for increased sensitivity, so the results of these studies presumably do not provide a realistic analysis of this test's effectiveness.

In our laboratory we have been evaluating the new Chlamydiazyme since March 1985. So far, of 680 cervical or urethral specimens tested by culture and by Chlamydiazyme, 117 have been positive for *Chlamydia* by one or both methods. Eighty-two were positive by both methods, 15 by culture only, and 20 by Chlamydiazyme only. For 2 of the 20 specimens reactive by Chlamydiazyme only, one or two elementary particles were seen on the accompanying Syva tests. The other 18 samples had low (< 0.5) absorbance, suggestive of possible false reactivity.

The laboratory performance of Chlamydiazyme is straightforward and easier to learn than the Syva test, which depends upon a final subjective opinion of the laboratory worker. However, the Chlamydiazyme does not lend itself well to the examination of only a few samples each day. It is not cost-effective to run less than 20 specimens in the Chlamydiazyme test. Therefore, this often causes a delay in reporting results, since samples must be held until enough are obtained to make a run worthwhile.

In summary, there is clearly a need for each individual laboratory to evaluate the advantages and disadvantages of these two commercial tests in relation to time, equipment, expertise, and work load before untertaking a commitment to using either one.

Lymphogranuloma Venereum

The serotype classification of *C. trachomatis* includes three groups of LGV organism: L-1, L-2, and L-3. While all organisms classified as *C. trachomatis* share the common biological property of forming inclusions that stain with iodine, the LGV serotypes differ considerably from other *C. trachomatis,* both in the laboratory and in human infections.

In the laboratory one characteristic difference between LGV and other *C. trachomatis* is that LGV can infect tissue culture cells without being centrifuged. Thus large amounts of LGV organisms can easily be prepared for research studies or antigen production; isolates can also conveniently be identified as LGV without resorting to serotyping. Also, other *Chlamydia* undergo only one replication cycle after infection because, in vitro, additional cells are not infected without intervening centrifugation; by contrast, LGV organisms will continue to lyse, infect adjoining cells, and replicate until no more cells are available. Thus it is necessary when working with LGV to stain cultures at specific times to avoid missing inclusions due to complete cell lysis. This natural high infectivity of LGV, combined with the ability of these organisms to survive for prolonged periods outside of cells, makes them good candidates to cross-contaminate other cell cultures. Accordingly, it is important when handling LGV in the laboratory either to be a biological hood or to work in an area physically removed from that where clinical specimens are processed for oculogenital *Chlamydia*.

In vivo, LGV organisms cause disease substantially different from that caused by trachoma (serotypes A-C) or oculogenital (serotypes D-K) strains of *C. trachomatis*. In men the common complaints of those seeking help for LGV infections are inguinal lymphadenopathy (buboes) and/or anorectal symptoms, while women usually present with anorectal infection. This means the laboratory that offers culture for LGV must be prepared to examine a variety of specimens, including urethral, cervical, and anorectal swabs, as well as lymph node aspirates.

Culture is not ordinarily used to diagnose LGV infection because this method has not been widely available. Another problem is that cultural diagnosis of LGV is not particularly sensitive. Although cultural isolation of the organism is the only certain way to identify LGV infection, sometimes growth in cell culture [62] or eggs [64] is not accomplished in patients with a distinct clinical picture of LGV, even when this is accompanied by good serologic confirmation.

The same criteria hold for developing a sensitive LGV culture system as have been mentioned for other *C. trachomatis* - proper samples, rapid transport, and quality control of the tissue culture system. Although LGV organisms will frequently grow in a tissue culture system that will not sustain other *Chlamydia,* complications brought by the clinical specimens may offset this advantage. Bubo aspirates may have a toxic effect on cell cultures and should be diluted with growth medium before inoculation; rectal specimens frequently contain heavy bacterial contamination that can destroy the cell monolayer. An original portion of each specimen for LGV culture should be stored frozen ($-70\,°C$); if cultures are lost to cell destruction then additional processing of the saved portion before retesting, addition of antibiotics, or further dilution may prove helpful.

In practice the diagnosis of LGV is generally made in the clinic on the basis of patient signs and symptoms, with laboratory confirmation sought by the use of CF testing. Although other serologic tests have been used for confirmation of LGV infection, including MIF [81] and counterimmunoelectrophoresis [8], these are not yet available to the average laboratory because of the complexity of antigen preparation. However, CF antigen is commercially available (*Institut für Mikrobiologie*, CH-9000 St. Gallen, Switzerland). This application of the CF test is the major justification for its persistence in chlamydiology, since it is not of much diagnostic value in oculogenital infections.

Schachter [64] has noted in his patient studies that recovery of LGV organisms by egg culture has always been accompanied by a concurrent CF titer. Titers greater than 64 are considered confirmatory for infection with LGV organisms. Titers less than this can be confusing and must be interpreted with great care. These have been considered indicative of cross-reactivity with oculogenital strains, but patients with low titers may also be infected with *C. trachomatis* LGV. Bolan et al. [6] isolated LGV serotype L-2 from the recta of three patients with acute proctitis; these titers ranged from 4 to 32.

Summary

As the number of clinical conditions attributable to sexually transmitted *C. trachomatis* infection increases, so too does the demand for identification of this widespread organism. At present, the most general, useful, and specific means of identification depends upon growth in tissue culture. Applied research directed at improving culture techniques can do much to make identification of this organism more widely available. Possible further areas of development include rapid means of identification of nonviable organisms, cell-free culture methods, and methods of attaining high infectivity of clinical specimens without centrifugation.

References

1. Amortegui AJ, Meyer MP (1985) Enzyme immunoassay for detection of *Chlamydia trachomatis* from the cervix. Obstet Gynecol 65: 523–526
2. Baselski V, McNeeley G, Ryan G, Robison M, Bry E (1984) A comparison of Chlamydiazyme t6 cell culture isolation for the detection of *C. trachomatis* in cervical swab specimens. Abstracts of annual ASM meeting, St Louis, C 108
3. Bennett AH, Hipp SS, Alford LA (1982) Pyosemia and carriage of *Chlamydia* and *Ureaplasma* in men. J Urol 128: 54–56
4. Berrón S, Vazquez J, Fenoll A (1984) Letter to the editor. Lancet 8394: 110
5. Bird BR, Forrester FT (1981) Laboratory diagnosis of *Chlamydia trachomatis* infections. US Department of Health and Human Services, Center for Disease Control, Atlanta

6. Bolan RK, Sands M, Schachter J, Miner RC, Drew WL (1982) Lymphogranuloma venereum and acute ulcerative proctitis. Am J Med 72: 703–706
7. Bruce AW, Chadwick P, Willett WS, O'Shaughnessy M (1982) Letter to the editor. J Urol 128: 156
8. Caldwell HD, Kuo EL (1977) Serologic diagnosis of lymphogranuloma venereum by counter-immunoelectrophoresis with a *Chlamydia trachomatis* protein antigen. J Immunol 118: 442–445
9. Cevenine E, Donati M, Rumpianesi F (1981) Elementary bodies as single antigen in a micro-ELISA test for *Chlamydia trachomatis* antibodies. Microbiologica 4: 347–351
10. Croy TR, Kuo CC, Wang SP (1975) Comparative susceptibility of 11 mammalian cell lines to infection with trachoma organisms. J Clin Microbiol 1: 434–439
11. Darouger S, Jones BR, Kinneson JR, Vaughn-Jackson JD, Dunlop EMC (1972) Chlamydial infection: advances in the diagnostic isolation of *Chlamydia,* including TRIC agent from the eye, genital tract and rectum. Br J Vener Dis 48: 416–420
12. Darougar S, Cubitt S, Jones BR (1974) Effect of high-speed centrifugation on the sensitivity of irradiated McCoy cell culture for the isolation of *Chlamydia.* Br J Vener Dis 50: 303–312
13. Darougar S, Woodland RM, Forsey T, Cubitt S, Allami S, Jones BR (1977) Isolation of *Chlamydia* from ocular infections. In: Hobson D, Holmes K (eds) Nongonococcal urethritis and related infections. American Society for Microbiology, Washington, pp 295–298
14. Evans RT (1980) Suppression of *Chlamydia trachomatis* inclusion formation by fetal calf serum in cycloheximide-treated McCoy cells. J Clin Microbiol 11: 424–425
15. Evans RT, Taylor-Robinson D (1979) Comparison of various McCoy cell treatment procedures used for detection of *Chlamydia trachomatis.* J Clin Microbiol 10: 198–201
16. Finn MP, Ohlin A, Schachter J (1983) Enzyme-linked immunosorbent assay for immunoglobulin G and M antibodies to *Chlamydia trachomatis.* J Clin Microbiol 17: 848–852
17. Gordon FB, Quan AL (1965) Isolation of the trachoma agent in cell culture. Proc Soc Exp Biol Med 118: 354–359
18. Gupta PK, Lee EF, Erozan YS, Frost JK, Geddes ST, Donovan PA (1979) Cytologic investigations in *Chlamydia* infection. Acta Cytol (Baltimore) 23: 315–320
19. Hall LF, Shayegani M, Hipp SS (1982) Genital infections of women: the role of the laboratory in identification of microorganisms associated with vaginitis. NY State J Med 82: 1317–1320
20. Hanna L (1977) Microscopic demonstration of chlamydial inclusions by Giemsa, iodine or immunofluorescence stains. In: Hobson D, Holmes K (eds) Nongonococcal urethritis and related infections. American Society for Microbiology, Washington, pp 266–271
21. Hanna L, Keshishyan H, Brooks GF, Stites DP, Jawetz E (1981) Effect of seminal plasma on *Chlamydia trachomatis* strains LB-1 in cell culture. Infect Immun 32: 404–406
22. Hawkins DA, Thomas BJ, Taylor-Robinson D (1984) Letter to the editor. Lancet 8393: 38
23. Henry-Suchet J, Loffredo V (1980) Chlamydiae and mycoplasma genital infection in salpingitis and tubal sterility. Lancet 1: 539
24. Henry-Suchet J, Catalin F, Loffredo V, Serfaty D, Siboulet A, Perol Y, Sanson MJ, Debache C, Pigeau F, Coppin R, deBrux J, Poynard T (1980) Microbiology of specimens obtained by laparoscopy from controls and from patients with PID or infertility with tubal obstruction: *Chlamydia trachomatis* and *Ureaplasma urealyticum.* Am J Obstet Gynecol 138: 1022–1025
25. Hilgarth von M, Ross A (1982) Chlamydien-Nachweis durch Vaginalzytologie. Fortschr Med 100: 391–392
26. Hipp SS, Kirkwood M, Gump DW (1980) Artifacts resembling *Chlamydia trachomatis.* N Engl J Med 302: 1367
27. Hipp SS, Kirkwood MW, Han Y (1983) Recovery of *Chlamydia trachomatis* by inoculation of McCoy cell suspensions. Current Microbiol 9: 141–144
28. Hipp SS, Rockwood L, White L, Lufkin D, Kirkwood M (1984) Antimicrobial activity of nine commercial vaginal products on *Chlamydia, Candida, Trichomonas* and *Ureaplasma.* Annals NY Acad Sci 435: 598–600
29. Hobson D (1977) Tissue culture procedures for the isolation of *Chlamydia trachomatis* from patients with gonococcal genital infections. In: Hobson D, Holmes K (eds) Nongonococcal urethritis and related infections. American Society for Microbiology, Washington, pp 286–295
30. Johannisson G, Lowhagen G, Lycke E (1980) Genital *Chlamydia trachomatis* infection in women. Obstet Gynecol 56: 671–675
31. Johnson FWA, Hobson D (1976) Factors affecting the sensitivity of replicating McCoy cells in the isolation and growth of chlamydia A (TRIC agents). J Hyg Camb 76: 441–451

32. Johnson FWA, Hobson D (1977) The effect of penicillin on genital strains of *Chlamydia tracho-matis* in tissue culture. J Antimicrob Chemother 3: 49-56
33. Jones MF, Smith TF, Houglum AJ, Hermann JE (1984a) Detection of *Chlamydia trachomatis* in genital specimens by the Chlamydiazyme test. Abstracts of annual ASM meeting, St Louis, C 104
34. Jones MF, Smith TF, Houglum AJ, Hermann JE (1984b) Detection of *Chlamydia trachomatis* in genital specimens by the Chlamydiazyme test. J Clin Microbiol 20: 465-467
35. Kordova N, Wilt JC, Sekla L, Wenman WM, Stackiw W, Feltham S (1982) New commercial chlamydial antigens in the serology of chlamydial infections in a selected population of the Province of Manitoba. Can J Public Health 73: 424-426
36. Krech T, Gerhard-Fsadni D, Hofmann N, Miller SM (1985) Letter to the editor. Lancet May 18, pp 1161-1162
37. Kuo CC, Wang SP, Wentworth BB, Grayson JT (1972) Primary isolation of TRIC organisms in HeLa 229 cells treated with DEAE-dextran. J Infect Dis 125: 665-668
38. Lamont HC, Nichols RL (1979) Immunology of chlamydial infections. In: Good R, Day S (eds) Comprehensive immunology, part I, pp 441-474
39. LaScolea LJ, Baldigo SM (1982) Infectivity of *Chlamydia trachomatis* in tissue culture with new-born calf serum. J Clin Microbiol 15: 951-953
40. LaScolea L, Keddell JE (1981) Efficacy of various cell culture procedures for detection of *Chlamydia trachomatis* and applicability to diagnosis of pediatric infections. J Clin Microbiol 13: 705-708
41. Leman C, Metzel P, Kurpiewski G (1984) Evaluation of Chlamydiazyme for the detection of *Chlamydia trachomatis* antigen in cervical specimens. Abstracts of annual ASM meeting, St Louis, C 103
42. Levy NJ, McCormack MW (1982) Detection of serum antibody to *Chlamydia* with ELISA. In: Mårdh PA, Holmes KK, Oriel JD, Piot P, Schachter J (eds) Chlamydial infections. Elsevier Biomedical, Amsterdam, pp 341-344
43. Lewis VJ, Thacker WL, Mitchell SH (1976) Enzyme-linked immunosorbent assay for chlamydial antibodies. J Clin Microbiol 6: 507-510
44. McComb DE, Puznizk CI (1974) Microcell culture method for isolation of *Chlamydia trachomatis*. Appl Microbiol 28: 727-729
45. Madin SH, Darby CF (1958) Established kidney cell lines of normal adult bovine and ovine origin. Proc Soc Exp Biol Med 98: 574-576
46. Mallinson H, Turner GC, Carey PB, Khan MH (1984) Letter to the editor. Lancet 8387: 1180
47. Mårdh PA, Weström L (1970) Tubal and cervical cultures in acute salpingitis with special reference to *Mycoplasma hominis* and T-strain mycoplasmas. Br J Vener Dis 46: 179-186
48. Mårdh PA, Zeeberg B (1981) Toxic effect of sampling swabs and transportation test tubes on the information of intracytoplasmic inclusions of *Chlamydia trachomatis* in McCoy cell cultures. Br J Vener Dis 57: 268-272
49. Mårdh PA, Ripa KT, Svensson L, Weström L (1977) *Chlamydia trachomatis* infection in patients with acute salpingitis. N Engl J Med 296: 1377-1379
50. Mårdh PA, Ripa KT, Colleen S, Treharne JD, Darougar S (1978) Role of *Chlamydia trachomatis* in non-acute prostatitis. Br J Vener Dis 54: 330-334
51. Mårdh PA, Colleen S, Sylwan J (1980) Inhibitory effect on the formation of chlamydial inclusions in McCoy cells by seminal fluid and some of its components. Invest Urol 17: 510-513
52. Osborn MF, Johnson AP (1982) Effect of various analgesics and lubricants on isolation of *Chlamydia trachomatis* and *Neisseria gonorrhoeae*. J Clin Microbiol 15: 522-524
53. Paavonen J (1979) *Chlamydia trachomatis*-induced urethritis in female partners of men with nongonococcal urethritis. Sex Transm Dis 6: 69-71
54. Paavonen J (1979) Chlamydial infections. Med Biol 57: 152-164
55. Quinn TC, Warfield P, Kappus E, Barbacci M, Spence M (1985) Screening for *Chlamydia trachomatis* infection in an inner-city population: a comparison of diagnostic methods. J Infect Dis 152: 419-423
56. Richmond SJ (1974) The isolation of *Chlamydia* subgroup A *(Chlamydia trachomatis)* in irradiated McCoy cells. Med Lab Technol 31: 7-9
57. Richmond SJ, Caul EO (1975) Fluorescent antibody studies in chlamydial infections. J Clin Microbiol 1: 345-352

58. Ridgeway GL, Moss V, Mumtaz G, Atia W, Emmerson AM, Oriel JD (1982) Provision of a chlamydial culture service to a sexually transmitted diseases clinic. Br J Vener Dis 58: 236–238

59. Ripa MT, Mårdh PA (1977) Cultivation of *Chlamydia trachomatis* in cycloheximide-treated McCoy cells. J Clin Microbiol 6: 328–331

60. Ruijs G, Kraai EJ, vanVoorst Vader PC, Schirm J, Schroeder FP (1984) Letter to the editor. Lancet 8383: 960

61. Saikku P, Paavonen J (1978) Single-antigen immunofluorescence test for chlamydial antibodies. J Clin Microbiol 8: 119–122

62. Schachter J (1981) Confirmatory serodiagnosis of lymphogranuloma venereum proctitis may yield false-positive results due to other chlamydial infections of the rectum. Sex Transm Dis 8: 26–28

63. Schachter J, Dawson CR (1978) Human chlamydial infections. PSG, Littleton, chapt 11

64. Schachter J, Smith DE, Dawson CR, Anderson WR, Deller JJ, Hoke AW, Smartt WH, Meyer KF (1969) Lymphogranuloma venereum. I Comparison of the Frei test, complement fixation test, and isolation of the agent. J Infect Dis 120: 372–375

65. Schachter J, Cles L, Ray R, Hines PA (1979) Failure of serology in diagnosing chlamydial infections of the female genital tract. J Clin Microbiol 10: 647–649

66. Schachter J, Grossman M, Azimi PH (1982) Serology of *Chlamydia trachomatis* in infants. J Infect Dis 146: 530–535

67. Shafer MA, Chew KL, Kromhout LK, Beck A, Sweet RL, Schachter J, King EB (1985) Chlamydial endocervical infections and cytologic findings in sexually active female adolescents. Am J Obstet Gynecol 151: 765–771

68. Smith TF (1977) Comparative recoveries of *Chlamydia* from urethral specimens using glass vials and plastic microtiter plates. Am J Clin Pathol 67: 496–498

69. Smith TF, Weed LA (1975) Comparison of urethral swabs, urine and urinary sediment for the isolation of *Chlamydia*. J Clin Microbiol 2: 134–135

70. Sompolinsky B, Richmond S (1974) Growth of *Chlamydia trachomatis* in McCoy cells treated with cytochalasin B. Appl Microbiol 28: 912–914

71. Stephens RS, Tam MR, Kuo C, Nowinski RC (1982) Monoclonal antibodies to *Chlamydia trachomatis:* antibody specificities and antigen characterization. J Immunol 128: 1083–1089

72. Tam MR, Stamm WE, Handsfield HH, Stephens R, Kuo C-C, Holmes KK, Ditzenberger K, Krieger M, Nowinski RC (1984) Culture-independent diagnosis of *Chlamydia trachomatis* using monoclonal antibodies. N Engl J Med 310: 1146–1150

73. Taylor HR, Rapoza PA, Kiessling LA, Quinn TC (1984) Letter to the editor. Lancet 8393: 38

74. Taylor-Robinson D, Hawkins DA, Thomas BJ (1985) Letter to the editor. J Clin Pathol 38: 236–237

75. Thomas BJ, Evans RT, Hutchinson GR, Taylor-Robinson D (1977) Early detection of chlamydial inclusions combining the use of cycloheximide-treated McCoy cells and immunofluorescence staining. J Clin Microbiol 6: 285–292

76. Tillotson JR (1981) Chlamydial trachomatis prostatitis: a presumptive case. NY State Dept of Health: IDI News No 2

77. Treharne JD (1982) *Chlamydia trachomatis:* serological diagnosis. Infection 10 [suppl 1]: S 25

78. Treharne JD, Darougar S, Jones BR (1977) Modification of the MIF test to provide a routine serodiagnostic test for chlamydial infection. J Clin Pathol 30: 510–517

79. Valvo JR, Caldamone AA, Emilson LBV, Hipp SS, Cockett ATK (1980) Alterations in seminal pH and leukocytes associated with T-mycoplasma (T-strains) and male infertility. Am College Surg, Surg Forum 31: 579–582

80. Wang S, Grayston JT (1970) Immunologic relationship between genital TRIC, lymphogranuloma venereum and related organisms in a new microtiter indirect immunofluorescence test. Am J Ophthalmol 70: 367–374

81. Wang S, Grayston JT (1974) Human serology in *Chlamydia trachomatis* infection with microimmunofluorescence. J Infect Dis 130: 338–397

82. Wentworth BB, Alexander ER (1974) Isolation of *Chlamydia trachomatis* by use of 5-iodo-2-deoxyuridine-treated cells. Appl Microbiol 27: 912–916

83. World Health Organization (1975) Guide to the laboratory diagnosis of trachoma. World Health Organization, Geneva, p 25

Genital Infections – Male

William R. Bowie

Division of Infectious Diseases, University of British Columbia, 910 W. 10th Avenue, Vancouver B.C. V5Z 1M9, Canada

Introduction

Chlamydia trachomatis infections in men, both alone and concurrent with infections by other pathogens, such as *Neisseria gonorrhoeae,* are important because they are frequent and because infected men are a major reservoir of disease in the community. Fortunately, in contradistinction to the case with chlamydial infections in women, severe complications are unusual in men. Furthermore, most men with symptoms can be treated appropriately without the need to make a specific diagnosis of chlamydial infection. Male genital disease due to serovars of *C. trachomatis* other than lymphogranuloma venereum (LGV) strains include asymptomatic urethral infection, nongonococcal urethritis, concurrent infection with *N. gonorrhoeae,* postgonococcal urethritis, epididymitis, symptomatic and asymptomatic proctitis, but not prostatitis. These strains also probably have a role in some cases of Reiter's syndrome (see chapter on Reiter's syndrome). LGV serovars produce LGV and proctitis.

Asymptomatic Urethral Infection

Initial studies on chlamydial infections in men, performed in sexually transmitted disease clinics, showed rates of isolation of *C. trachomatis* of 35%–45% from men with nongonococcal urethritis, 30% from men with urethral gonorrhea, and 0–5% from men without obvious urethritis [1–3]. More recent studies have accentuated the importance of asymptomatic infection in men. In a study of male United States military personnel, 11 of 97 men without symptoms had *C. trachomatis* isolated from the urethra [4]. Only two (18%) of the infected men had pyuria; this is similar to the 9% rate of pyuria detected in uninfected men. The only feature that differentiated infected men from uninfected men was a history of urethritis (six of 11 versus 15 of 86, $p < 0.02$). Studies in Sweden have shown that male contacts of women with proven genital *C. trachomatis* infection are frequently asymptomatically infected [5]. Among 95 male contacts of women with proven genital *C. trachomatis* infection, *C. trachomatis* was isolated from 50 (53%). The infection was asymptomatic in 50%. For comparison purposes, among 265 male contacts of women with gonorrhea, 171 (78%) were infected with *N. gonorrhoeae,* but again 50% were asymptomatic.

Chlamydial Infections
Edited by P. Reeve
© Springer-Verlag Berlin Heidelberg 1987

The observation that *C. trachomatis* urethral infection is often asymptomatic is not surprising. The generally milder illness caused by *C. trachomatis* (as compared to gonococcal urethritis), the tendency of men with nongonococcal urethritis to ignore symptoms longer than men with gonorrhea, and the ability of *C. trachomatis* to produce a long-term infection almost made the finding inevitable. Asymptomatic infection in men presents a major problem because the men (a) remain sexually active because they do not know that they are infected; (b) would not normally consult health care personnel; and (c) would not be recognized as having infection unless culture samples were taken. Without culture their infection would only be identified if infection was identified in a partner. It is likely that long-term persistence of chlamydial urethritis is frequent, but good prospective data are lacking. Such men are definitely at risk of developing symptomatic urethritis, epididymitis, or sexually acquired reactive arthritis.

Male Urethritis

Urethritis can conveniently be divided into gonococcal and nongonococcal urethritis, on the basis of the presence or absence of *N. gonorrhoeae*. The distinction is very helpful clinically and therapeutically, but does not provide information about the presence or absence of *C. trachomatis* in a specific individual. That is, although 25%–60% (usually 30%–40%) of men with acute untreated nongonococcal urethritis, 5%–35% (usually 20%) of heterosexual men with urethral gonorrhea, and 5% of homosexual men with urethral gonorrhea have urethral *C. trachomatis* infection, in a specific person there are no clinical characteristics that indicate whether or not *C. trachomatis* is present.

The evidence supporting *C. trachomatis* as a primary cause of urethritis is overwhelming. It includes isolation results summarized above; serologic studies in carefully selected populations (see below); better response of chlamydial urethritis than of urethritis in which *C. trachomatis* is not identified, when treatment is initiated with antimicrobials having better activity against *C. trachomatis* than other potential pathogens; isolation studies from female partners which show that rates of isolation of *C. trachomatis* are higher in contacts of men from whom *C. trachomatis* is isolated than in contacts of men from whom *C. trachomatis* is not isolated; follow-up in untreated patients, which shows persistence of *C. trachomatis;* prospective follow-up of men with gonorrhea and concurrent *C. trachomatis* who do not receive therapy that will eradicate *C. trachomatis* (see below); and primate inoculations which result in urethral infection. These data have been extensively reviewed [6]. The serologic data in a highly selected group of men with nongonococcal urethritis who had had relatively few sex partners and no prior history of urethritis indicated that *C. trachomatis* was a primary cause of urethritis [7]. Of ten men with positive urethral cultures for *C. trachomatis* and symptoms for 10 or fewer days, nine had no microimmunofluorescent antibody to *C. trachomatis* in acute sera, but had it detected in convalescent sera. However, the possibility still lingers that in some cases *C. trachomatis* infection, or at least isolation of *C. trachomatis,* may be precipitated by other infections. This possibility was proposed by Richmond and Clarke in 1977 [8], in part because in some series rates of isolation of *C. trachomatis* were similar in men with nongonococcal urethritis and urethral gonorrhea [3], and development of post-gonococcal urethritis is an obvious example of a situation where a chlamydial infection follows a gonococcal infection. More recently, Oriel and Ridgway, in a study of female contacts of men with nongonococcal urethritis or gonorrhea, found that the rate of isolation of *C. trachomatis* from the female was dependent both upon the rate of isolation of *C. trachomatis* from the men and also on active infection of the female with *N. gonorrhoeae* [9]. These observations are compatible with two opposing conclusions. That is, presence of *C. trachomatis* could make an individual more susceptible to *N. gonorrhoeae,* or else *N. gonorrhoeae* could reactivate quiescent or subclinical *C. trachomatis* infection. The correct explanation is not yet known and thus the possibility that some *C. trachomatis* genital infections are reactivated rather than newly acquired must be considered.

An intriguing question is the role of *C. trachomatis* in the 60% of acute untreated cases of nongonococcal urethritis and the over 95% of cases of persistent or recurrent nongonococcal urethritis which have negative cultures for *C. trachomatis*. With all the methodological problems inherent in isolating *C. trachomatis,* it is not surprising that some culture-negative cases are probably due to *C. trachomatis*. In fact, this may occur in approximately 10% of cases, even under optimal conditions [7]. There are clearly other causes. *Ureaplasma urealyticum* is a significant cause of many of these *C. trachomatis* culture-negative cases, but 20%–30% of cases of acute nongonococcal urethritis are culture negative for both *C. trachomatis* and *U. urealyticum*. These cases respond less well than C. trachomatis culture-positive cases to antimicrobials active against *C. trachomatis* [7]. In summary, it is very unlikely that active infection with *C. trachomatis* is a cause of many of the cases with negative cultures for *C. trachomatis*. However, a host response to amounts of chlamydial antigens that are not detectable by current techniques remains a possible explanation for some of these cases. This possibility will be very hard to prove or disprove.

Gonorrhea and Postgonococcal Urethritis

C. trachomatis is frequently present in men and women with gonorrhea. When they are treated with spectinomycin or single-dose penicillin therapy, the *C. trachomatis* infection is not usually eradicated and persistence of *C. trachomatis* infection usually leads to development of symptomatic urethritis in the ensuing weeks. This is called postgonococcal urethritis. The delay between the onset of gonorrhea and the development of postgonococcal urethritis is presumed to be due to differences in incubation periods of the different pathogens, but it is possible that the gonococcal infection reactivates a subclinical chlamydial infection in some cases. Postgonococcal urethritis is in most ways similar to a nongonococcal urethritis, except that the rate of isolation of *C. trachomatis* tends to be higher, although rates of isolation are quite variable in different published studies. The rates ranged from 15% to 81% in nine studies conducted from 1972 to 1978. In the combined series, 141 (50%) of 282 men with postgonococcal urethritis had *C. trachomatis* isolated. Postgonococcal urethritis tends to arise 1 or more weeks after treatment of gonorrhea. In practical terms this means that men could be inappropriately reassured that everything is normal at the postgonorrhea test of cure evaluation.

In contrast to the high rates of development of postgonococcal urethritis after penicillins, postgonococcal urethritis is infrequent in men treated with tetracycline 500 mg orally four times daily for 5 days or trimethoprim-sulfamethoxazole 9 tablets (720-3600 mg) once daily for 3 days [10].

Epididymitis

Many bacteria, fungi, parasites, and yeasts have been implicated as causes of acute or chronic epididymitis. However, until appropriately designed studies looking for multiple agents including sexually transmitted pathogens were performed, 55%-100% of cases of acute epididymitis were considered to be idiopathic. More recent studies have clearly shown that C. trachomatis is a major cause of acute epididymitis in populations at risk of acquiring sexually transmitted diseases, whereas classic urinary tract pathogens such as coliforms and Pseudomonads are important causes in older men, men with structural abnormalities of the urinary tract, and probably homosexuals.

Frequent coexistence of urethritis in men with acute epididymitis was well known. In 1977, Harnisch et al. [11] first convincingly demonstrated the importance of C. trachomatis in acute epididymitis. Among 24 men with acute epididymitis seen in 1972-1973, four of six men over 45 years of age had coliforms or Pseudomonads isolated, whereas among 18 men under 32 years of age, C. trachomatis was found in six, gonorrhea in six, and both in one. In 1979, Berger et al. expanded this series to a total of 50 men with symptoms of less than 2 months' duration, in association with tenderness and swelling maximal in the epididymis [12]. Nineteen of the men had epididymal aspirates cultured as well as urethral and urine specimens. Overall, coliform of Pseudomonas infection was diagnosed in 12 of 16 men over 35 years of age and in one of 34 men under the age of 35. Escherichia coli was isolated from the epididymis of six out of six men with coliform infection versus none or ten without. N. gonorrhoeae or C. trachomatis infection was diagnosed in one of 16 over 35 and in 24 of 34 under 35 years of age. C. trachomatis was isolated from five epididymal aspirates, in association with positive cultures from the urethra in three cases and with a positive semen culture in one case.

Most clinical and historical features were of little help in differentiating between the 13 patients with coliforms, seven with N. gonorrhoeae, 17 with C. trachomatis, and 13 with other or unknown etiologies [12]. However, all men with gonorrhea had copious urethral discharge, whereas others did not. A lesser amount of discharge was present in 11 of 17 with C. trachomatis, three of 13 with other etiologies, and two of 13 men with coliform infection (both with catheters). Compared with men in whom coliforms were causing the epididymitis, men with C. trachomatis had a tendency toward more inguinal pain (eight of 17 versus two of 13). Preexisting genitourinary pathology was present only in the group with coliform or Pseudomonas infections, where seven of 13 had abnormalities. Gram-negative intracellular diplococci were present in the urethral smears from all seven men with gonorrhea.

All men with *Pseudomonad* or coliform infection had over one gram-negative rod per oil immersion field in the gram stain of one drop of uncentrifuged urine.

In addition to these studies in humans, a grivet monkey model supports the role of *C. trachomatis* as a cause of epididymitis: inoculation of *C. trachomatis* into the spermatic cord was followed by inflammation and swelling.

Proctitis

Lymphogranuloma venereum has been known since 1936 to involve the rectum. That non-LGV serovars of *C. trachomatis* could infect the recta of women was recognized soon after cell culture techniques for isolation of *C. trachomatis* were systematically utilized. The rate of isolation of *C. trachomatis* from the recta of heterosexual men has not been evaluated, but is presumed to be negligible or nonexistent. However, *C. trachomatis* is isolated from a proportion of homosexual men with proctocolitis, and LGV serovars especially may be associated with particularly severe disease.

In a study by Quinn et al. in Seattle, *C. trachomatis* was isolated from the recta of 24 (8.3%) of 288 male homosexuals in a sexually transmitted disease clinic [13]. Rates of isolation were 12% from men with symptoms of proctitis and 6% from men without symptoms. All men with symptoms and all but one man without practiced passive rectal intercourse. Fecal leukocytes were present in rectal gram stains from all men with symptoms and 85% of men without. As with urethritis, infection was often mixed. Other rectal pathogens were present in four of 11 men with symptoms and 21% of men without symptoms.

Disease associated with non-LGV serovars tended to be relatively mild. Symptoms included mild to moderate rectal discharge, pain, and diarrhea. At anoscopy and sigmoidoscopy, the mucosa was erythematous or friable. Biopsies revealed a polymorphonuclear leukocyte infiltrate within the lamina propria. Three of the 24 isolates were L2 strains. With these strains disease was more severe clinically, and at sigmoidoscopy the mucosa was friable and there were extensive hemorrhages and ulcerations. Biopsies in two of the three men showed diffuse inflammation with crypt abscesses, granulomas, and giant cells, consistent with Crohn's disease.

Prostatitis

Although the data have not been extensively evaluated, there is no convincing evidence that *C. trachomatis* is a cause of acute prostatitis. In contrast, the etiology of chronic nonbacterial prostatitis and prostatodynia remains unknown in the majority of cases. The observation that some men with these conditions respond to treatment with tetracyclines, erythromycin, or trimethoprim-sulfamethoxazole, antimicrobials that should be active against *C. trachomatis,* and the failure to detect other pathogens are consistent with the possibility that *C. trachomatis* could be a cause. However, *C. trachomatis* is thought not to infect glandular tissue, and thus the prostate would be an unexpected site to become infected. So far, studies have not supported *C. trachomatis* as a cause of nonbacterial prostatitis [14]. Failure to identify *C. trachomatis* infection does not, however, exclude the possibility that the disease is in part caused by a hypersensitivity reaction to *C. trachomatis*. Since such a mechanism contributes to the manifestation of trachoma in some situations, it is at least conceivable that it could be associated with development of prostatitis. The preliminary studies by Ballard et al. showing that men with chronic nonbacterial prostatitis were significantly more likely than controls to show positive delayed hypersensitivity skin test reactions to *C. trachomatis* and the apparent clinical improvement and reduction in the skin test response on erythromycin therapy are consistent with this possibility [15].

Lymphogranuloma Venereum

Lymphogranuloma venereum is the only *C. trachomatis* infection that regularly produces multisystem involvement and constitutional manifestations. It has a primary phase with a transient lesion, a secondary stage with suppurative regional lymphadenopathy and prominent constitutional symptoms, and a late phase with sequelae related to fibrotic changes and abnormal lymphatic drainage. LGV is endemic in Asia, Africa, and South America, but as many as 500 cases per year have been reported in the United States since 1965. Many of these are based on low-titer complement fixation seropositivity and cannot be confirmed by microimmunofluorescence testing. In the United States, LGV is reported three times as frequently in men as in women, with the highest occurrence being in persons of low socioeconomic status living in the southeast, in male homosexuals, and in persons returning from regions outside the United States where it is endemic. Transmission by fomites, laboratory accidents, and nonsexual contact has been reported, but LGV is primarily sexually transmitted. The reservoirs are not certain, but probably are persons with asymptomatic or ignored symptomatic urethral, cervical, or anorectal infection.

Three days to 3 weeks after exposure, a small, painless, herpetiform vesicle or a nonindurated papule or ulcer develops on the penis in one-third or less of infected men. Because the lesion heals quickly, does not scar, and antedates the lymphadenopathy, LGV is not usually diagnosed at this stage. In homosexual men, a primary anorectal rather than a primary genital infection may occur. With anorectal infection, the initial manifestations may be diarrhea, tenesmus, and bloody or mucopurulent anal discharge associated with diffuse or discrete ulcerations in the rectosigmoid colon.

A recent study conducted in Swaziland and South Africa described a different presentation of LGV [16]. Isolates of *C. trachomatis,* presumed but not proved to be LGV, were recovered from genital ulcers of ten men and two women. Most had microimmunofluorescence antibody to *C. trachomatis*. Inguinal lymphadenopathy was present in only 50%, was usually unilateral, and was fluctuant in only one. The lesions were unlike the typically described transient lesion. They were deep, measured 4–6 mm in diameter, had elevated edges, and had a purulent or indurated base. The mean duration of illness was 72 days, with a median of 45 days.

In typical LGV, 2-6 weeks after initial exposure, regional lymphadenopathy develops. The location varies with the initial site of involvement: inguinal and femoral nodes with penile and occasionally anal infection, and hypogastric and deep iliac nodes with anorectal infection. The most characteristic manifestation is the inguinal syndrome, with unilateral or bilateral (one-third of cases) painful inguinal lymphadenopathy frequently associated with palpable iliac and femoral nodes on the ipsilateral side. The nodes are initially discrete, but because of the extensive periadenitis, the nodes become matted and the overlying skin becomes fixed and inflamed. Pathologically, the nodes initially show characteristic small stellate abscesses surrounded by histiocytes. The abscesses eventually coalesce, becoming necrotic and fluctuant. The overlying skin thins, and the nodes eventually suppurate to form multiple draining fistulas. The fistulas heal over a period of several months, but scars and masses persist. Complications at this stage include anal fistula, perirectal abscesses, and rectovesical and ischiorectal fistulas secondary to suppuration associated with anorectal infection.

Systemic symptoms are usually present in the second stage. Fever, chills, anorexia, headache, meningismus, myalgias, and arthralgias are common. Less common are aseptic meningitis, meningoencephalitis, conjunctivitis, hepatitis, erythema nodosum, and arthritis with a sterile effusion. Leukocytosis, elevated erythrocyte sedimentation rate, and abnormal liver function tests are common. Hyperglobulinemia, increased IgA, IgG, and IgM, rheumatoid factor, and mixed cryoglobulins have been reported. In addition, positive serologic tests for syphilis have been reported, but in these patients the diagnosis of syphilis should be strongly considered.

Disease may progress, or complications may develop in a third stage. Approximately 5% of the men with LGV have chronic and progressive ulcerative or infiltrative involvement of the penis, urethra, or scrotum with fistulas, ulcers, and urethral strictures that especially involve the posterior urethra. Late complications can also arise secondary to fibrosis and abnormal lymphatic drainage. Rectal strictures 2-6 cm from the anal orifice may develop. Polypoid swelling of the skin and keloid formation in the genitalia in association with induration and lymphedema may clinically resemble granuloma inguinale and genital tuberculosis. Uncommonly, the induration and lymphedema may produce genital elephantiasis with enlargement of the penis.

Manifestations of Infection

The repertoire of the responses of the genital tract to infection is limited. With respect to the urethra, inflammation can be shown as discharge or meatal inflammation, and symptoms include discharge, burning on urination, or an itch experienced at the end of the urethra or in the urethra. The differences between gonorrhea and either nongonococcal urethritis or postgonococcal urethritis are quantitative rather than qualitative, and apply to comparisons of groups rather than to individuals. Thus with gonorrhea, discharge tends to be more acute, profuse, and purulent, whereas in men with nongonococcal urethritis it is often gradual in onset, less obvious, and mucoid. With respect to likelihood of chlamydial infection being present,

however, these differences are helpful only in that men with postgonococcal urethritis and nongonococcal urethritis are more likely to have C. trachomatis infection
than men with gonorrhea. At the time a man is initially seen there is no clinical way
of differentiating types of urethritis into those that do or do not involve C. trachomatis.

Among men with urethritis due to C. trachomatis, symptoms of frequency, ur-
gency, nocturia, hematuria, perineal pain, pain with bowel movements, scrotal
swelling, inguinal lymphadenopathy, genital rash, chills, and fever are all very unusual and if present suggest other or concurrent infections. Urethritis is often present in men with epididymitis, but epididymitis is an infrequent complication of
urethritis. History of diarrhea, conjunctivitis, arthralgias or arthritis, and skin or oral
lesions suggest the possibility of Reiter's syndrome or reactive arthritis.

Of major concern for diagnosis and control of chlamydial (and also gonococcal)
infection is asymptomatic or minimally symptomatic urethritis. It has been well
demonstrated that the diagnosis of urethritis in men with symptoms may be missed
without optimal examination. Among several studies where men presented to sexually transmitted disease clinics with symptoms suggestive of urethritis, but a firm diagnosis could not be established on the initial visit, almost one-half had definite
urethritis (usually nongonococcal urethritis) when examined in the morning prior to
voiding. Thus when urethritis is suspected but cannot be proved, the patient should
be reexamined in the morning prior to voiding.

The whole genital region should be carefully examined. For detection of urethritis, the urethra should be stripped from the base to the meatus three or four times to
express discharge if it is not present spontaneously. Increased numbers of polymorphonuclear leukocytes are almost always present with green, yellow, or white discharge and are usually present with mucoid discharge. Clear discharge, especially
following treatment, often does not have increased numbers of polymorphonuclear
leukocytes. Typically, in men with nongonococcal urethritis a discharge is only noted in the morning. However, on examination later in the day, staining may be noted
on underwear even if it cannot be detected directly.

Manifestations associated with epididymitis, proctitis, and LGV were discussed
previously.

Laboratory Diagnosis

The appropriate techniques for obtaining, transporting, and culturing specimens for
C. trachomatis are discussed in the chapter entitled "Laboratory Diagnosis of
Chlamydial Infection". However, when the clinician first examines the patient, the
specific microbiological data will not be known, and potential syndromes must be
recognized. There are two main principles that must always be remembered. The
first is the importance of an optimal examination as discussed previously. The second is that as many as possible of the potential etiologies of the presenting syndrome should be specifically sought. For urethritis, this usually means N. gonorrhoeae and C. trachomatis. For epididymitis this means testing for the presence of
pathogens in the urine and epididymis if feasible, as well as for urethral pathogens.

For proctocolitis it means testing for enteric bacterial pathogens, parasites, herpes-virus, *Treponema pallidum, N. gonorrhoeae,* and *C. trachomatis.*

With the exception of LGV, serology is usually not helpful in diagnosis of geni-tal chlamydial infections in men because of the high background level of microim-munofluorescent antibody to *C. trachomatis* antigens, at least in sexually transmit-ted disease clinic populations. The usefulness of serologic evaluation in other populations requires more evaluation. In men with LGV, complement-fixing anti-bodies showing a fourfold increase in titer or a single titer of 1:64 or greater are very suggestive. High microimmunofluorescent antibody titers to one of the LGV sero-vars are more sensitive and more specific than complement-fixing antibody. Use of the Frei test to detect a cellular immune response to chlamydial antigens is neither sensitive nor specific using currently available antigens.

Confirmation of urethritis requires demonstration of increased numbers of polymorphonuclear leukocytes in urethral material. Since gonococcal and chlamy-dial infection can be present without an increased number of polymorphonuclear leukocytes, it is obvious that absence of a polymorphonuclear leukocyte response does not exclude infection, but demonstration of its presence allows initiation of a management plan for the patient and partners. A polymorphonuclear leukocyte re-sponse can be detected either in a smear of endourethral material or exudate if pre-sent, or in the sediment of the first voided urine. Ideally, the patient should not have voided for 4 or more hours, and preferably overnight if the patient has symptoms but few or no clinical findings. A mean of four or more polymorphonuclear leuko-cytes per field in five oil immersion ($\times 1000$) fields on smear, or the presence of 15 or more polymorphonuclear leukocytes in two or more of five fields in the sediment of the first 10 ml urine, correlates with the presence of urethritis [17, 18].

To detect polymorphonuclear leukocytes in urine, after as long an interval with-out voiding as feasible, the first 10–15 ml urine voided should be collected and cen-trifuged at 400 g for 10 min. All but 0.5 ml of the supernatant is decanted and the sediment is resuspended in the residual urine. Sufficient sediment is placed on a slide to cover approximately 1 cm^2 and a coverslip is placed over it. The area under the coverslip is examined at a magnification of $\times 400$, and the number of polymor-phonuclear leukocytes in each of five fields is enumerated. To obtain material for gram stain, a swab of urethral exudate can be obtained when obvious discharge is present, but when discharge is minimal or absent a calcium alginate urethrogenital swab should be inserted into the urethra 1–2 cm proximal to the fossa navicularis. The swab is then rolled gently back and forth over a glass slide to cover an area of approximately 1 cm^2. The slide is then gram stained and the gram-stained specimen is scanned at magnification of $\times 100$. Areas that have the largest numbers of poly-morphonuclear leukocytes are then examined under oil ($\times 1000$) and the number of polymorphonuclear leukocytes in each of five fields is recorded. While polymor-phonuclear leukocytes are being enumerated the slide should also be examined for gram-negative diplococci. This provides the most rapid and least expensive means of differentiating gonococcal from nongonococcal urethritis. For experienced mic-roscopists, the sensitivity and specificity of typical gram-negative intracellular di-plococci as indicating gonorrhea and increased numbers of polymorphonuclear leukocytes without any evidence of typical or atypical gram-negative displococci as indicating nongonococcal urethritis are close to 100% in sexually transmitted disease clinic populations [19]. In situations with a lower prevalence of gonorrhea, the specificity may be lower. When the gram-stained specimen is interpreted as being equivocal, or when an individual with expertise is not available to interpret the gram stain, cultures are necessary. Cultures are also necessary for treatment failures, if penicillinase-producing *N. gonorrhoea* are prevalent or are suspected on epidemiologic grounds, and for test for cure.

Management

Once chlamydial infection is diagnosed, or a syndrome potentially caused by *C. trachomatis* is identified, choice of an antimicrobial regimen that will reliably eradicate *C. trachomatis* is easy. Although there are differences in methodology between the many studies evaluating efficacy of antimicrobials against urethral *C. trachomatis*, studies consistently show that 7 days of a tetracycline will usually eradicate *C. trachomatis*. The differences in study design deserve further emphasis because they assume major importance when new or potentially suboptimal regimens are evaluated. Clearly, all studies require cultures before and after treatment, because there are numerous examples where there is clinical improvement despite persistence or recurrence of *C. trachomatis*. The major difference between studies is in the duration of follow-up after treatment. A short follow-up, for example a week after treatment, is easier for the investigator because it takes less time, fewer patients default from the study, and patients are less likely to receive other medications or resume having intercourse with new or untreated partners. Longer follow-up increases the time commitments of the investigator and patients and increases the risk of confounding influences. Nevertheless, in the author's opinion longer follow-up, for at least 4-6 weeks after treatment, is necessary. In two recent studies by the author, one-third of men with *C. trachomatis* urethritis had recurrence of *C. trachomatis* on suboptimal regimens (erythromycin stearate 250 mg four times daily for 7 days, clindamycin 600 mg three times daily for 7 days) [20]. Microbiological recurrence with no evidence of pyuria and microbiological recurrence more than 2 weeks after treatment were frequent. Such failures would not have been recognized without the longer follow-up in conjunction with cultures.

Numerous studies have shown that tetracycline 250 mg or 500 mg four times daily for 7 days or minocycline or doxycycline 100 mg once or twice daily for 7 days will reliably eradicate *C. trachomatis* from the urethra (summarized in reference 20). Results with erythromycin are less satisfactory in men [20]. Erythromycin stearate 250 mg four times daily for 7 days was associated with recurrence of *C. trachomatis* in 13 of 35 men. Erythromycin 500 mg twice daily for 10 days failed to eradicate it from five of 23 men. However, erythromycin 500 mg twice daily for 2 weeks has usually been successful. It is presumed that erythromycin 500 mg four times daily for 7 days will eradicate *C. trachomatis*, but more data are required. Sulfisoxazole 500 mg four times daily for 10 days reliably eradicates *C. trachomatis* as well. Less experience is available with trimethoprim-sulfamethoxazole, and it is likely that only the sulfonamide portion is active. Rifampin 600 mg once daily for 6 days was highly active in one study. Both penicillins and clindamycin, when given in high oral doses for prolonged periods, frequently eradicate *C. trachomatis*, but not reliably. Aminoglycosides, metronidazole, and newer cephalosporins are not active in vitro and probably are not active in vivo. Thus 7 days of a tetracycline or erythromycin and 10 days of a sulfonamide will usually eradicate *C. trachomatis*. However, this does not necessarily mean that the patient will be cured. This is an important concept which often confuses clinicians, who are surprised when patients with chlamydial urethritis have persistent or recurrent urethritis, even though *C. trachomatis* is eradicated. Numerous studies have shown that persistent or recurrent urethritis arises in 15%–20% of men with nongonococcal urethritis who initially have *C. trachomatis* isolated and then eradicated. This presumably occurs because of concurrent presence of other pathogens, or the host response to infection.

The statistical likelihood of concurrent pathogens being present actually determines which of available antimicrobials should be utilized. For male urethritis, the coexisting pathogens are likely to be *N. gonorrhoeae* or *U. urealyticum*, and a tetracycline is the usual drug of choice. Because of ease of administration, the preferred regimen is doxycycline 100 mg orally twice daily for 7 days, but tetracycline 500 mg four times daily for 7 days is likely to be equally active and is less expensive [21]. These regimens are the treatment of choice for asymptomatic urethritis, nongonococcal urethritis, postgonococcal urethritis, and proctitis due to *C. trachomatis*. The author also strongly believes that they should be used to treat uncomplicated gonorrhea, in conjunction with a standard single-dose penicillin, spectinomycin, or cefoxitin regimen. Some might feel that use of a regimen active against *C. trachomatis* is not needed for treatment of gonorrhea in homosexual men because of low rates of concurrent urethral *C. trachomatis*. However, in an ongoing study in Vancouver, 5% of homosexual men with gonorrhea had *C. trachomatis* in the urethra and another 6% had *C. trachomatis* in the rectum, so that overall 11% had *C. trachomatis* infection. Erythromycin 500 mg (but not 250 mg) four times daily should reliably eradicate *C. trachomatis* and usually eradicates *U. urealyticum* (including the 10% of isolates resistant to tetracyclines), but is not reliable against *N. gonorrhoeae*. Overall, it is probably as effective as tetracyclines for nongonococcal urethritis, but would not be the drug of choice if used alone for gonorrhea or urethritis which has not been evaluated by laboratory testing to differentiate between gonococcal and nongonococcal urethritis. Sulfonamides are not used for treatment of the above syndromes because of lack of activity against *U. urealyticum* and *N. gonorrhoeae*.

The antimicrobial treatment of complicated chlamydial infections in men is also simple. For chlamydial epididymitis, or epididymitis arising in sexually active heterosexual men without coliforms having been identified in the urine or epididymal aspirates, doxycycline 100 mg twice daily or tetracycline 500 mg four times daily should be administered for at least 10 days. For genital, inguinal, or anorectal LGV, at least 2 weeks of antimicrobials should be given, with the options in decreasing order of preference being tetracycline 500 mg four times daily, doxycycline 100 mg twice daily, erythromycin 500 mg four times daily, and a sulfonamide such as sulfisoxazole 500 mg four times daily.

Besides antimicrobial treatment of the patient, it is critically important to evaluate and then treat sexual partners with similar regimens, even if they are asymptomatic. Because infection in women is less likely to be recognized by the syndromic approach, yet sequelae are more severe, this part cannot be stressed too highly. An examination of the partner that appears to be "normal" but which does not include genital cultures for *C. trachomatis* does not rule out the need for treatment of the partner. Patients should refrain from having sexual intercourse until the partner has been adequately treated. The need for follow-up examination in asymptomatic men who take their medications properly is minimal, because even if urethritis is present, *C. trachomatis* will not be. Men with persistent or recurrent symptoms should be carefully reevaluated. Among compliant men with urethritis at follow-up, those who did not resume sexual intercourse or only had intercourse with an adequately treated partner almost never have *C. trachomatis* reisolated. In contrast, men who were not compliant, received suboptimal regimens (especially of erythromycin), or were exposed to new or untreated partners occasionally did have *C. trachomatis* reisolated. If available, repeat cultures for *C. trachomatis* are indicated in this group. Men who have symptoms at follow-up should be carefully questioned about compliance with respect to medications and resumption of sexual activity; should be carefully examined to detect other, less usual causes of urethritis, such as warts or herpesvirus; and should have the presence of urethritis confirmed by detection of increased numbers of polymorphonuclear leukocytes. If no other cause is found, or if *U. urealyticum* is isolated at follow-up in the presence of urethritis, then treatment should be given with erythromycin 500 mg four times daily for 2 weeks if a tetracycline was used first, or with a tetracycline regimen if an erythromycin regimen was used first.

Patients with epididymitis may require bedrest with elevation of the scrotum, analgesics, and ice packs to the scrotum. Patients with LGV should have the buboes aspirated on one or more occasions if they become fluctuant.

References

1. Dunlop EMC, Vaughan-Jackson JD, Darougar S, Jones BR (1972) Chlamydial infection. Incidence in "non-specific" urethritis. Br J Vener Dis 48: 425–428
2. Oriel JD, Reeve P, Powis P, Miller A, Nicol CS (1972) Chlamydial infection. Isolation of chlamydia from patients with non-specific genital infection. Br J Vener Dis 48: 429–436
3. Richmond SJ, Hilton AL, Clarke SKR (1972) Chlamydial infection. Role of chlamydia subgroup A in non-gonococcal and post-gonococcal urethritis. Br J Vener Dis 48: 437–444
4. Podgore JK, Holmes KK, Alexander ER (1982) Asymptomatic urethral infections due to *Chlamydia trachomatis* in male U.S. military personnel. J Infect Dis 146: 828
5. Thelin I, Wennstrom A-M, Mårdh P-A (1980) Contact-tracing in patients with genital chlamydial infection. Br J Vener Dis 56: 259–262
6. Schachter J (1978) Chlamydial infections. N Engl J Med 298: 428–435, 490–495, 540–549
7. Bowie WR, Wang S-P, Alexander ER, Floyd J, Forsyth PS, Pollock HM, Lin J-SL, Buchanan TM, Holmes KK (1977) Etiology of nongonococcal urethritis. Evidence for *Chlamydia trachomatis* and *Ureaplasma urealyticum*. J Clin Invest 59: 735–742
8. Richmond SJ, Clarke SKR (1977) Problems in assigning a causative role to chlamydiae isolated in nongonococcal urethritis. In: Hobson D, Holmes KK (eds) Nongonococcal urethritis and related infections. American Society for Microbiology, Washington, pp 43–46
9. Oriel JD, Ridgway GL (1982) Studies of the epidemiology of chlamydial infection of the human genital tract. In: Mårdh P-A, Holmes KK, Oriel JD, Piot P, Schachter J (eds) Chlamydial infections. Elsevier Biomedical, New York, pp 425–428
10. McCabe ME, Fiumara NJ, McCormack WM (1981) Effect of three regimens for the treatment of gonorrhea on the incidence of postgonococcal urethritis. Presented at the 1st sexually

transmitted diseases world congress, San Juan, Puerto Rico, 15-21 November 1981, abstract 130

11. Harnisch JP, Berger RE, Alexander ER, Monda G, Holmes KK (1977) Aetiology of acute epididymitis. Lancet 1: 819-821

12. Berger RE, Alexander ER, Harnisch JP, Paulsen CA, Monda G, Ansell J, Holmes KK (1979) Etiology, manifestations and therapy of acute epididymitis: prospective study of 50 cases. J Urol 121: 750-754

13. Quinn TC, Goodell SE, Mkrtichian E, Schuffler MD, Wang S-P, Stamm WE, Holmes KK (1981) *Chlamydia trachomatis* proctitis. N Engl J Med 305: 195-200

14. Mårdh P-A, Ripa KT, Colleen S, Treharne JD, Darougar S (1978) Role of *Chlamydia trachomatis* in non-acute prostatitis. Br J Vener Dis 54: 330-334

15. Ballard RC, Koornhof HJ, Mausenbaum E, van Blerk PJ (1981) The role of *Chlamydia trachomatis* in the aetiology of chronic prostatitis and treatment of the condition with erythromycin. Presented at the 12th international congress of chemotherapy, Florence, 1981, abstract 223

16. Piot P, Ballard RC, Fehler HG, van Dyck E, Ursi JP, Meheus AZ (1982) Isolation of *Chlamydia trachomatis* from genital ulcerations in Southern Africa. In: Mårdh P-A, Holmes KK, Oriel JD, Piot P, Schachter J (eds) *Chlamydial infections*. Elsevier Biomedical, New York, pp 115-118

17. Bowie WR (1978) Comparison of gram stain and first-voided urine sediment in the diagnosis of urethritis. Sex Transm Dis 5: 39-42

18. Swartz SL, Kraus SJ, Herrmann KL, Stargel MD, Brown WJ, Allen SD (1978) Diagnosis and etiology of nongonococcal urethritis. J Infect Dis 138: 445-454

19. Jacobs NF, Kraus SJ (1975) Gonococcal and nongonococcal urethritis in men. Clinical and laboratory differentiation. Ann Intern Med 82: 7-12

20. Bowie WR (1982) Treatment of chlamydial infections. In: Mårdh P-A, Holmes KK, Oriel J, Piot P, Schachter J (eds) *Chlamydial infections*. Elsevier Biomedical, New York, pp 231-244

21. Centers for Disease Control (1982) Sexually transmitted disease: treatment guidelines, 1982. Rev Infect Dis 4: S729-S746

Chlamydia Trachomatis:
Antibiotic Sensitivity and Chemotherapy

Walter E. Stamm

Division of Infectious Diseases, Department of Medicine, Harborview Medical Center, 325 Ninth Avenue, Seattle, WA 98104, USA

Introduction

Physicians initiate antibiotic treatment of presumed chlamydial infection for one of several reasons. Most often, recognition of a clinical syndrome known to be associated with *Chlamydia,* such as nongonococcal urethritis (NGU) [1] or mucopurulent cervicitis [2], leads to treatment. In this circumstance, treatment cannot be regarded as specific, since *Chlamydia* causes only 40%–50% of cases of NGU [1] and only 30%–40% of cases of mucopurulent cervicitis [2]. Treatment of the sexual contacts of men with NGU or women with mucopurulent cervicitis results in other patients with chlamydial infections being given antibiotics. Again, treatment in this instance, although warranted by the high prevalence of infection in these groups [3, 4], cannot be regarded as specific. The frequent coexistence of chlamydial infection in patients with gonorrhea has led to recommendations that heterosexual patients with gonorrhea be given antibiotic treatment that will also be effective against *Chlamydia* [5]. And finally, although *Chlamydia* cultures are not yet widely available, some patients are identified on the basis of a positive screening culture rather than by the presence of signs and symptoms. Screening of high-risk populations suggests that at least one-third of infected men and probably the majority of infected women can be identified only by screening cultures [6–9].

These considerations imply that, in most patients, the physician initiates treatment for chlamydial infection without benefit of microbiologic confirmation, and also manages the patient without subsequent proof of cure. They also indicate that, in the absence of cultures, many patients with asymptomatic or minimally symptomatic chlamydial infections do not receive appropriate treatment. It is to be hoped that technological advances will make *Chlamydia* cultures and/or other diagnostic tests more widely available in the future, making treatment for *Chlamydia* more specific and less empiric [10].

Chlamydial Infections
Edited by P. Reeve
© Springer-Verlag Berlin Heidelberg 1987

In Vitro Evaluation of Antimicrobials Against *C. trachomatis*

In vitro evaluation of an antimicrobial's activity against *C. trachomatis* utilizing infected cell culture systems has proved valuable in predicting the efficacy of antibiotics in subsequent treatment trials. Methods of in vitro evaluation vary from laboratory to laboratory in procedural details such as type of cell line used, number of inclusion-forming units in the initial inoculum, duration and force of centrifugation, the time at which antibiotics are added to the cell culture system, the method used for staining inclusions, and the definition employed for the end point of an antibiotic's effectiveness [11–17]. Despite these methodological variations, the reported minimal inhibitory concentration or MIC (usually defined as the lowest concentration of antibiotic that prevents the formation of inclusions) for most antibiotics falls within a relatively narrow range (Table 1). To date, no evidence of geographic variation in antimicrobial sensitivity of *C. trachomatis* has been demonstrated. Likewise, strain to strain variation and immunotype-related variability in antimicrobial sensitivity have not been described.

Reported in vitro studies indicate that antimicrobials with consistently high activity against *C. trachomatis* include the tetracyclines (doxycycline, minocycline, and tetracycline hydrochloride); the macrolides (erythromycin, rosaramicin, spiramycin); rifampicin; and the sulfonamides. Despite the fact that tetracyclines are widely used in humans for the treatment of both chlamydial and other infections, and are added to animal feeds as growth promoters, in vitro resistance to tetracy-

Table 1. In vitro activity of selected antimicrobials against *Chlamydia trachomatis*

	Johannisson et al.	Bowie et al.	Kuo et al.	Blackman et al.	Ridgway et al.
Penicillin		9.6→38	0.1 (>100)[a]	0.25→1.0	1.0
Ampicillin		0.5→4	0.1 (>100)[a]		0.25
Pivampicillin	0.25				
Tetracycline	0.1	0.06	0.02–0.5	0.5	0.03
Minocycline		0.03			0.03
Doxycycline	0.05	0.03			0.03
Naladixic acid		>64			
Rosoxacin		4			
Streptomycin	>100	>10000			
Gentamicin	>100	>1000			>512
Spectinomycin	>100	125–250			64
Erythromycin	0.5	0.25–0.5	0.1–0.5	0.25–0.5	0.6
Metronidazole		>5000			>256
Rifampin		0.008		0.06	0.007
Vancomycin	>100				>256
Trimethoprim	>100				128
Sulfamethoxazole	50		2–200		4.0
TMP-SMX	25				
Clindamycin		1.0			1.0
Chloramphenicol			10		4.0

[a] MIC for viability (in parentheses) differed from MIC for infectivity by a factor of 5 or more.

cline has not been reported for *C. trachomatis*. In our laboratory, in vitro assessment of tetracycline resistance in 22 strains obtained from men and women with uncomplicated genital infection who were found to be *Chlamydia* positive 10–21 days following treatment with tetracycline showed that all were sensitive to ≤ 0.3 µg/ml of tetracycline hydrochloride. Thus reinfection, poor compliance, or inadequate dose and/or duration of treatment usually explains apparent drug failure in such patients, not resistance to tetracycline. Low-level resistance to erythromycin (MIC = 0.6 µg/ml) has been reported in a single *C. trachomatis* strain [18], but has not been related to treatment failure or relapse. In vitro resistance to sulfonamides has been noted, and resistance to rifampicin can easily be produced in vitro [19] but has not been described in the few patients treated for chlamydial infections with this drug. Although plasmids have been demonstrated in *Chlamydia* [20], none has been shown to confer antimicrobial resistance as yet.

Antimicrobials with little or no apparent in vitro activity against *C. trachomatis* include the aminoglycosides, the aminocyclitols (spectinomycin), nalidixic acid, trimethoprim, vancomycin, metronidazole, lincomycin and the cephalosporins including the newer third-generation agents. Most of the penicillins, (penicillin G, ampicillin, amoxicillin, pivampicillin, and cloxacillin) exhibit intermediate activity against *Chlamydia*, producing alterations in the number and shape of inclusions at relatively low concentrations but not totally preventing inclusion formation until high concentrations (Table 1). Clindamycin and chloramphenicol both have reported MICs that also fall in an intermediate range.

Clinical Evaluation of Antimicrobials in C. trachomatis Infections

General Considerations

As with other sexually transmitted infections, evaluation of the effectiveness of treatment regimens for *C. trachomatis* is complicated by a number of factors. First, patients may be reinfected by untreated sex partners, so that relapse and reinfection are often difficult to distinguish. Second, poor patient compliance (especially with the multiple dose and 7–14 day regimens required for chlamydial infections) rather than actual antimicrobial ineffectiveness probably explains some apparent treatment failures. Third, many genital pathogens produce similar clinical syndromes, and when more than one is present in the same patient, the elimination of one pathogen may not result in clinical cure. Thus the clinical and microbiological responses to a given treatment regimen may not always concur. Fourth, selection of a treatment regimen for presumed chlamydial infection must take into account both possible coexisting infections (e.g., synchronous gonorrhea and chlamydial infection) and possible alternative etiologies (e.g., *Ureaplasma urealyticum* infection in men with NGU). Since treatment for most common genital syndromes such as urethritis or cervicitis is usually prescribed without specific cultures being obtained, the ideal treatment regimen should be effective not only against *Chlamydia* but also against other pathogens that may produce indistinguishable clinical syndromes. Finally, about two-thirds of chlamydial infections in women and at least a quarter of those in men produce few or no symptoms [6–9]. Such patients can obviously be recognized only through culture screening or by contact investigation initiated upon discovery of an infected sex partner. The high proportion of *Chlamydia*-infected patients who lack specific symptoms and signs of infection, coupled with the relative unavailability of *Chlamydia* cultures, makes examination and empirical treatment of sex partners of men with NGU and women with mucopurulent cervicitis and salpingitis critical.

Treatment of *C. trachomatis* Infections in Men

Most clinical evidence regarding the effectiveness of various antimicrobials against *C. trachomatis* has been accumulated in men with urethritis (Table 2) [21–32]. Two general principles have emerged from these studies: penicillin, ampicillin, amoxicillin, cephalosporins, and spectinomycin in single-dose regimens given for treatment

Table 2. Summary of selected studies evaluating oral antimicrobial treatment of *Chlamydia trachomatis* urethritis in men

Reference	Regimen	Efficacy[a]
31	Tetracycline 500 mg four times a day for 7 days	35/35 (100%)
24	Erythromycin stearate 500 mg every 12 h for 2 wks	30/31 (97%)
25	Doxycycline 200 mg for 2 days and 100 mg for 12 days	50/52 (96%)
22	Triple tetracycline every day for 7 days Triple tetracycline every day for 21 days	11/12 (92%) 16/16 (100%)
41	Minocycline 200 mg immediately, 100 mg twice a day for 6 days Rifampin 600 mg every day for 6 days	39/40 (98%) 52/53 (98%)
27	Erythromycin 500 mg every 12 h for 15 days Lymecycline 300 mg every 12 h for 10 days Lymecycline 300 mg every 12 h for 20 days	27/30 (90%) 21/24 (88%) 18/21 (86%)
11	Pivampicillin 750 mg three times a day for 7 days	19/22 (86%)
47	Doxycycline 200 mg for 1 day, 100 mg for 6 days TMP-SMX (160/800 mg) twice a day for 10 days Erythromycin 500 mg twice a day for 10 days	56/57 (98%) 18/20 (90%) 18/23 (78%)
29	Trimethoprim-sulfadiazine (160/500 mg) 1 tab twice a day for 14 days	18/19 (95%)
32	Tetracycline 250 mg four times a day for 7 days Tetracycline 500 mg four times a day for 7 days Rosaramicin 250 mg four times a day for 7 days	21/24 (88%) 33/36 (92%) 38/42 (90%)
26	Amoxicillin 750 mg three times a day for 10 days	6/6 (100%)

[a] Studies cited in Tables 2 and 3 performed *Chlamydia* cultures before, just after, and 2–3 weeks following completion of treatment; efficacy as expressed in the tables

$$= \frac{\text{Patients with negative Chlamydia cultures on visit 2 and visit 3}}{\text{Patients returning for follow-up visits 2 and 3}}$$

Eradication of *Chlamydia* was usually, but not always, associated with clinical resolution of signs and symptoms.

of gonorrhea usually do not eradicate concomitant chlamydial infection; and 7 or more days of treatment with the tetracyclines or macrolides eradicates *C. trachomatis* from nearly all men, at least as determined by short-term follow-up. However, chlamydial infection recurs 3–6 weeks after treatment in 5%–10% of these men and cannot clearly be designated as reinfection or relapse. Most such recurrences are of the same immunotype as the original infecting strain [4], and nearly all cause recurrent clinical evidence of urethritis. In addition, despite elimination of *C. trachomatis,* 10%–15% of men develop persisting or relapsing symptoms, perhaps due to simultaneous infection with another agent.

In men with NGU, trials using either placebos or agents such as spectinomycin which are ineffective against *C. trachomatis* have clearly established the greater effectiveness of specific antimicrobial treatment both in eliminating signs and symptoms of infection and in eradicating *Chlamydia* [29, 30]. Clinical trials indicate that 7–10 days of oral tetracycline hydrochloride, doxycycline, minocycline, triple tetracycline, erythromycin, trimethoprim-sulfamethoxazole, sulfonamides, and rosaramicin all achieve comparable clinical cure rates of approximately 85%–95% in men with chlamydial NGU (Table 2). Somewhat lower cure rates with erythromycin than with tetracycline have been observed, but a recent multicenter study comparing the two drugs found no difference in efficacy against *C. trachomatis* [33]. Although relatively ineffective against *C. trachomatis* in vitro and when administered as a single dose, amoxicillin, when given as 750 mg orally three times a day for 10 days, apparently eliminated *Chlamydia* from six men with NGU followed up for 24–48 days [26]. Pivampicillin gave similar results in high dosage [11]. Although symptoms usually subsided as cultures became negative in these studies, the possibility cannot be excluded that subclinical chlamydial infection persisted after amoxicillin or pivamicillin treatment.

Because it is effective, well tolerated, and cheap, tetracycline hydrochloride has been the most widely used regimen for treatment of NGU. The recommended length of therapy ranges from 7 to 21 days. In two studies in which 7 days of tetracycline or minocycline were compared with 21 days of therapy with these drugs, however, no difference was found [22, 23]. Thus prolongation of tetracycline therapy beyond 1 week appears unnecessary, provided sex partners can be treated concurrently.

Antimicrobial treatment of the two major complications of chlamydial urethritis in men, epididymitis and Reiter's syndrome, has been little studied. Early treatment of chlamydial urethritis with tetracycline may prevent Reiter's syndrome, but the effect of tetracycline therapy on established Reiter's syndrome has not been well studied. Men with either idiopathic epididymitis or proven chlamydial epididymis should receive tetracycline hydrochloride 500 mg orally twice a day for 10 days or doxycycline 100 mg twice a day for 10 days. In small treatment trials, ampicillin 3.5 g followed by 500 mg orally four times a day appeared less effective than tetracycline in these patients [35, 36]. In another trial, the clinical response to doxycycline in men with acute epididymitis was excellent [37].

Proctitis

Recent studies of small numbers of patients indicate that tetracycline hydrochloride, 500 mg orally four times a day for 7 days, effectively treats symptomatic chlamydial proctitis in either homosexual men or heterosexual women [38, 39]. Proctitis due to lymphogranuloma venereum (LGV) strains of *C. trachomatis,* recognizable by its more severe clinical course [38], should probably be treated with 14 days of tetracycline hydrochloride, 2 g daily. Shorter durations of treatment have not been adequately studied, nor have drugs other than tetracycline.

Lymphogranuloma Venereum

The clinical syndrome of classic LGV (painful inguinal buboes, fever, and transient genital ulceration) occurs rarely in the industrialized world but more frequently in tropical countries. Older treatment trials without cultural confirmation of infection gave rise to recommendations for treatment that included 21 days of a tetracycline or a sulfonamid. A recent study by Perine et al. in patients with proven LGV demonstrated a satisfactory clinical response to 7–14 days of tetracycline or TMP-SMX [40].

Infections in Women

Cervicitis and Urethritis
Fewer studies have assessed the treatment of chlamydial cervical infection in women than have evaluated treatment of NGU in men (Table 3). Available studies suggest that 7–14 days of tetracycline, minocycline, doxycycline, erythromycin, sulfonamides, or TMP-SMX effectively eliminate *C. trachomatis* from the cervix, at least through 3 weeks of follow-up [41–50]. Clinical signs of mucopurulent cervicitis resolve coincident with cultures becoming negative. Longer treatment regimens using these drugs have been equally effective and have no apparent advantage over 7–10 days of treatment. Regimens shorter than 7 days have been little studied. Ripa et al. treated five women with two doses of 240/1200 mg TMP-SMX given 5 h apart, and found all five to be culture negative 14 days later [51]. During pregnancy, erythromycin 250 mg orally four times a day for 7 days or sulfisoxazole 500 mg orally four times a day for 10 days should be used for treatment of chlamydial cervicitis, but the effectiveness of these regimens has not been well established.

Simultaneous chlamydial infection of the urethra can be demonstrated in the majority of women with chlamydial cervical infection, and some women have urethral infection without positive cervical cultures [52]. Chlamydial urethritis may present clinically as dysuria, frequency, and sterile pyuria (the acute urethral syndrome) [53]. A small, double-blind, placebo-controlled study showed that women with symptomatic chlamydial urethritis given doxycyline 100 mg orally twice a day for 10 days experienced resolution of their clinical symptoms and pyuria more quickly than those given placebo [54]. Although not specifically evaluated as yet,

Table 3. Summary of selected studies evaluating antimicrobial treatment of *Chlamydial trachomatis* cervicitis

Reference	Regimen	Efficacy	
45	Triple tetracycline 300 mg twice a day for 7 days	20/20	(100%)
24	Oxytetracycline 250 mg four times a day for 14 days	49/50	(98%)
44	Oxytetracycline 250 mg four times a day for 21 days	145/161	(90%)
27	Erythromycin 500 mg twice a day for 15 days	13/17	(76%)
	Lymecycline 300 mg twice a day for 10 days	18/20	(90%)
	Lymecycline 300 mg twice a day for 20 days	14/14	(100%)
46	Doxycycline 200 mg immediately, 100 mg twice a day for 8 days	10/10	(100%)
29	Trimethoprim-sulfadiazine (160/500); 1 tab twice a day for 14 days	15/15	(100%)
	Doxycycline 100 mg twice a day for 10 days	15/15	(100%)
47	Doxycycline 200 mg immediately, 100 mg twice a day for 9 days	55/58	(95%)
	Erythromycin 500 mg twice a day for 10 days	36/39	(92%)
	TMP-SMX (160/800 mg) 1 tab a day for 10 days	37/40	(93%)
48	Tetracycline 500 mg four times a day for 7 days	6/6	(100%)
	Tetracycline 250 mg four times a day for 7 days	6/6	(100%)
	Rosaramicin 250 mg four times a day for 7 days	9/11	(82%)
	Erythromycin 250 mg four times a day for 7 days	10/10	(100%)
49	Tetracycline 500 mg four times a day for 7 days	21/22	(95%)
	Erythromycin 250 mg four times a day for 7 days	12/12	(100%)
	Sulfisoxazole 500 mg four times a day for 10 days	8/8	(100%)

most of the treatment regimens effective for cervical infection are probably effective for urethral infection also.

Salpingitis, Endometritis, Perihepatitis
Few data regarding the efficacy of various antibiotic regimens in women with proven chlamydial salpingitis are available. In part, this is due to the difficulty in establishing the diagnosis microbiologically unless both cervical and tubal cultures are obtained. In a cooperative trial in the United States, tetracycline 500 mg orally four times a day for 10 days was no more effective than ampicillin 3.5 g + 1.0 g probenecid followed by 500 mg orally four times a day for 10 days in patients with nongonococcal pelvic inflammatory disease (PID) [55]. Of 52 women with PID proved by laparoscopy (one-half with *Chlamydia* isolated from the cervix before therapy), Gjonnaess et al. reported a 98% clinical response rate with lymecycline 300 mg orally daily for 14 days [56]. Gjonnaess also demonstrated a 95% cure rate in 334 women with PID given doxycycline, vs an 85% cure rate in 75 women given ampicillin ($p < 0.005$) [57]. Further comparative therapeutic studies in women with PID in whom comprehensive microbiological studies have been carried out are clearly needed. Until such data are available, most experts favor inclusions of at least one drug that is effective against *Chlamydia* in vitro in any treatment regimen for salpingitis, especially nongonococcal salpingitis. Doxycycline 100 mg orally twice a day or tetracycline 500 mg orally four times a day for 10-14 days are currently recom-

mended [5]. These regimens have also been successfully used in the small number of culturally confirmed cases of chlamydial endometritis and perihepatitis reported in the literature [58-60]. Treatment trials of patients with these less common syndromes have not been reported.

Treatment of Neonatal Infections

Neither silver nitrate ocular prophylaxis nor a single instillation of erythromycin ophthalmic ointment prevents chlamydial neonatal conjunctivitis [61]. Established chlamydial conjunctivitis should be treated with systemic rather than topical therapy because the latter is ineffective in eradicating eye infection and has no effect on concomitant nasopharyngeal infection [62]. Optimal therapy for neonatal inclusion conjunctivitis has not been established, but current studies support the use of erythromycin (40 mg/kg per day).

Studies of antibiotic treatment of infant pneumonia due to *Chlamydia* show that most patients can be cured with 150 mg sulfisoxazole per kilogram per day or 40 mg erythromycin per kilogram per day for 14-21 days [63]. Lower doses (30 mg/kg per day or less) of erythromycin, however, may be inadequate [64, 65].

Conclusions

Several groups of antibiotics, specifically the tetracyclines, macrolides, sulfonamides, and rifampin, exhibit excellent activity against *C. trachomatis* in vitro and have demonstrated efficacy in clinical trials. The clinical value of antibiotics with lesser in vitro activity against *C. trachomatis* (penicillins, clindamycin, some cephalosporins) needs further study, but preliminary trials suggest they may have some clinical efficacy when given for a week or more. Treatment of chlamydial infections generally requires at least 7 days of antibiotics, although shorter regimens have not been widely tested. In patients with synchronous gonorrhea and chlamydial infection, single-dose ampicillin, amoxicillin, or penicillin is ineffective against *Chlamydia*, while 3 days of TMP-SMX and 5 days of tetracycline appear to be effective [66].

Selection of an antibiotic for treatment of possible *C. trachomatis* infection is usually empirical rather than being based on a known positive culture. Since other microorganisms also cause syndromes indistinguishable clinically from those due to *Chlamydia*, choice of an antibiotic must be based upon the susceptibilities of these other pathogens as well. Thus tetracyclines provide activity not only against *Chlamydia* but also against most strains of gonococci, *U. urealyticum*, and *M. hominis*, although increasing tetracycline resistance has been reported for each of these three organisms. Tetracyclines also have activity against Enterobacteriaceae and against some anaerobes, which may be of importance in treating salpingitis. Macrolides possess excellent in vitro activity against *C. trachomatis*, *U. urealyticum*, and most gonococci, but not against *M. hominis*. Despite in vitro results, erythromycin effects an unacceptably low rate of cure of *N. gonorrhoeae*, and in some studies has apparently been less effective than tetracyclines against *Chlamydia*. Sulfonamides (including TMP-SMX) have excellent activity in vitro and in vivo against *C. trachomatis* and *N. gonorrhoeae,* but no activity against *M. hominis* or *U. urealyticum.* In pregnancy, sulfonamides (except in late pregnancy) and erythromycin are the drugs of choice for *C. trachomatis* infection. Further clinical studies are needed, especially assessing treatment of salpingitis, neonatal infections, and infections in pregnancy.

References

1. Schachter J (1978) Chlamydial infections. N Engl J Med 298: 428
2. Paavonen J, Brunham RC, Kiviat N, Stevens C, Kuo CC, Stamm WE, Holmes KK (1982) Cervicitis - etiologic, clinical, and histopathologic findings. In: Mårdh PA, Holmes KK, Oriel JD, Piot P, Schachter J (eds) Chlamydial infections. Elsevier Biomedical, Amsterdam, pp 141-147
3. Thelin I, Wennstrom A-M, Mårdh PA (1980) Contact tracing in patients with genital chlamydial infection. Br J Vener Dis 56: 259
4. Holmes KK, Handsfield HH, Wang SP, et al (1975) Etiology of nongonococcal urethritis. N Engl J Med 292: 1199
5. Sexually transmitted diseases treatment guidelines - 1982. Morbidity Mortality Weekly Report - Supplement 31: 335-625
6. Stamm WE, Koutsky LA, Benedetti JK, Jourden JL, Brunham RB, Holmes KK (1984) *Chlamydia trachomatis* urethral infections in men: prevalence, risk factors, and clinical manifestations. Ann Intern Med 100: 47-51
7. Podgore JK, Holmes KK, Alexander ER (1982) Asymptomatic urethral infections due to *Chlamydia trachomatis* in male US military personnel. J Infect Dis 146: 828
8. Richmond SJ, Paul ID, Taylor PK (1980) Value and feasibility of screening women attending STD clinics for cervical chlamydial infections. Br J Vener Dis 56: 92
9. Brunham R, Irwin B, Stamm WE, Holmes KK (1981) Epidemiological and clinical correlates of *C. trachomatis* and *N. gonorrhoeae* infection among women attending an STD clinic. Clin Res 29: 47A
10. Stamm WE, Holmes KK (1981) Chlamydia infections. What should we do while waiting for a diagnostic test. West J Med 135: 226-229
11. Johannison G, Sernryd A, Lycke E (1979) Susceptibility of *Chlamydia trachomatis* to antibiotics in vitro and in vivo. Sex Transm Dis 6: 50-57
12. Bowie WR, Lee CK, Alexander ER (1978) Prediction of efficacy of antimicrobial agents in treatment of infections due to *Chlamydia trachomatis.* J Infect Dis 138: 655-659
13. Bowie WR (1981) In vitro activity of clindamycin against *Chlamydia trachomatis.* Sex Transm Dis 8: 220-221
14. Bowie WR (1982) Lack of in vitro activity of cefoxitin, cefamandole, cefuroxime, and piperacillin against *Chlamydia trachomatis.* Antimicrob Agents Chemother 21: 339-340
15. Kuo CC, Wang SP, Grayston JT (1977) Antimicrobial activity of several antibiotics and a sulfonamide against *Chlamydia trachomatis* organisms in cell culture. Antimicrob Agents Chemother 12: 80-83
16. Blackman HJ, Yoneda C, Dawson CR, et al. (1977) Antibiotic susceptibility of *Chlamydia trachomatis.* Antimicrob Agents Chemother 12: 673-677
17. Ridgway GL, Owen JM, Oriel JD (1978) The antimicrobial susceptibility of *Chlamydia trachomatis* in cell culture. Br J Vener Dis 54: 103-106
18. Mourad A, Sweet RL, Sugs N, et al (1980) Relative resistance to erythromycin in *Chlamydia trachomatis.* Antimicrob Agents Chemother 18: 696-698
19. Jones RB, Ridgway GL, Boulding S, Hunley KL (1983) In vitro activity of rifamycins alone and in combination with other antibiotics against *Chlamydia trachomatis* - Rev Infect Disease 5: S 556-S 561
20. Lovett M, Kuo CC, Holmes KK, Falkow S (1980) Plasmids of the genus *Chlamydia.* In: Nelson JD, Grassi C (eds) Current chemotherapy and infectious diseases. American Society for Microbiology, Washington DC

21. Oriel JD, Reeve P, Thomas BJ, Nicol CS (1975) Infection with *Chlamydia* group A in men with urethritis due to *Neisseria gonorrhoeae*. J Infect Dis 131: 376
22. Thambar IV, Simmons PD, Thin RN, Darougar S, Yearsley P (1979) Double-blind comparison of two regimens in the treatment of NGU. Br J Vener Dis 55: 284
23. Bowie WR, Alexander ER, Floyd JF, Stimson JB, Holmes KK (1981) Therapy for nongonococcal urethritis double-blind randomized comparison of two doses and two durations of minocycline. Ann Intern Med 95: 306
24. Oriel JD, Ridgway GL, Tchamouroff S (1977) Comparison of erythromycin stearate and oxytetracycline in the treatment of non-gonococcal urethritis. Scott Med J 22: 375
25. Perroud HM, Vulliemin JF (1978) L'hyclate de doxycycline dans le traitment des urétrites non-gonococciques. Schweiz Med Wochenschr 108: 412
26. Bowie WR, Alexander ER, Holmes KK (1981) Eradication of *Chlamydia trachomatis* from the urethras of men with NGU by treatment with amoxicillin. Sex Transm Dis 8: 79
27. Lassus A, Paavonen J, Kousa M, Saikku P (1979) Erythromycin and lymecycline treatment in *Chlamydia*-positive and *Chlamydia*-negative nongonococcal urethritis. A partner-controlled study. Acta Derm Venereol (Stockh) 59: 278
28. Lassus A, Paavonen J, Kousa M, Saikku P (1979) Erythromycin and lymecycline treatment of *Chlamydia*-positive and *Chlamydia*-negative NGU - a partner-controlled study. Acta Derm Venereol (Stockh) 59: 278
29. Paavonen J, Kousa M, Saikku P, Vartianinen E, Kanerva L, Lassus A (1980) Treatment of NGU with trimethoprim-sulphadiazine and with placebo. A double blind partner controlled study. Br J Vener Dis 56: 101
30. Bowie WR, Alexander ER, Floyd JF, et al. (1976) Differential response of chlamydial and ureaplasma-associated urethritis to sulphafurazole (sulfisoxazole) and aminocyclitols. Lancet 2: 1276
31. Handsfield HH, Alexander ER, Wang SP, Pederson AHB, Holmes KK (1976) Differences in the therapeutic response of chlamydia-positive and chlamydia-negative forms of nongonococcal urethritis. J Am Vener Dis Assoc 2: 5
32. Stamm WE, Holmes KK (1980) Comparison of rosaramicin and tetracycline for the treatment of NGU. In: Nelson JD, Grassi C (eds) Current chemotherapy and infectious diseases. American Society of Microbiology, Vol 2, p 1274
33. Alexander ER, Harrison HR, McCormick WM, et al. (1982) Comparison of erythromycin and tetracycline for the treatment of nongonococcal urethritis in men. In: Mårdh PA, Holmes KK, Oriel JD, Piot P, Schachter J (eds) Chlamydial infections. Elsevier Biomedical, Amsterdam
34. Bowie WM (1982) Treatment of chlamydial infections. In: Mårdh PA, Holmes KK, Oriel JD, Piot P, Schachter J (eds) Chlamydial infections. Elsevier Biomedical, Amsterdam
35. Holmes KK (1979) Acute epididymitis. Curr Therap Res 26: 732-737
36. Berger RE, Alexander ER, Harnish JP, Paulsen CA, Monda GD, Ansell J, Holmes KK (1979) Etiology, manifestations, and therapy of acute epididymitis: prospective study of 50 cases. J Urol 121: 750
37. Nilsson T, Fischer AB (1979) Acute epididymitis. Curr Therap Res 26: 738-744
38. Stamm WE, Quinn TC, Mkrtichian EE, Wang SP, Schuffler MD, Holmes KK (1982) *Chlamydia trachomatis* proctitis. In: Mårdh PA, Holmes KK, Oriel JD, Piot P, Schachter J (eds) Chlamydial infections. Elsevier Biomedical, Amsterdam, pp 111-114
39. Quinn TC, Goodell SE, Mkrtichian E, Schuffer MD, Wang SP, Stamm WE, Holmes KK (1981) *Chlamydia trachomatis* proctitis. N Engl J Med 305: 195
40. Perine PL, Anderson AJ, Krause DW, et al. (1979) Diagnosis and treatment of LGV in Ethiopia. In: Proceedings of the 11th international congress of chemotherapy. American Society for Microbiology, pp 1280-1282
41. Coufalik ED, Taylor-Robinson D, Csonka GW (1979) Treatment of nongonococcal urethritis with rifampicin as a means of defining the role of *Ureaplasma urealyticum*. Br J Vener Dis 55: 36
42. Johannison G (1981) Studies on *Chlamydia trachomatis* as a cause of lower urogenital tract infection. Acta Derm Venereol (Stockh) Suppl 93
43. Oriel JD, Ridgway GL (1980) Comparison of erythromycin and oxytetracycline in the treatment of cervical infection by *Chlamydia trachomatis*. J Infect 2: 259-262
44. Rees E, Tait IA, Hobson D, Johnson FWA (1977) Chlamydia in relation to cervical infection

and pelvic inflammatory disease. In: Hobson D, Holmes KK (eds) Nongonococcal urethritis and related infections. American Society for Microbiology, Washington DC, p 67

45. Waugh MA, Nayyar KC (1977) Triple tetracycline (Deteclo) in treatment of chlamydial infection of the female genital tract. Br J Vener Dis 53: 96

46. Ripa KT, Svensson L, Mårdh PA, Weström L (1978) *Chlamydia trachomatis* cervicitis in gynecologic patients. Obstet Gynecol 52: 698

47. Bowie WR, Manzon LM, Borrie-Hume CJ, et al. (1982) Efficacy of treatment regimens for lower urogenital *Chlamydia trachomatis* infection in women. Am J Obstet Gynecol 142: 125–129

48. Brunham RC, Stamm WE, Washton H, Kuo CC, Stevens C, Holmes KK (1981) Rosaramicin, erythromycin and tetracycline in the treatment of urogenital infection with *Chlamydia trachomatis* in women. Abstracts of the 12th international congress of chemotherapy, Florence

49. Bowie WR (1980) Seven to ten day antimicrobial regimens for *Chlamydia trachomatis* cervical infection. Clin Res 28: 43A

50. Hunter J, Smith IW, Macauley A, Peutherer JF (1979) Response to treatment of chlamydial infection of uterine cervix. Lancet 2: 848

51. Svennson L, Westrom L, Mårdh PA (1981) *Chlamydia trachomatis* in women attending a gynecological outpatient clinic with lower genital tract infection. Br J Vener Dis 57: 259–262

52. Paavonen J (1979) *Chlamydia trachomatis*-induced urethritis in female partners of men with nongonococcal urethritis. Sex Transm Dis 6: 69

53. Stamm WE, Wagner K, Amsel R, Alexander ER, Turck M, Counts GW, Holmes KK (1980) Causes of the acute urethral syndrome in women. N Engl J Med 303: 409

54. Stamm WE, Running K, McKevitt M, Counts GW, Turck M, Holmes KK (1981) Treatment of the acute urethral syndrome. N Engl J Med 304: 956

55. Thompson S, Holcomb G, Cheng S, et al. (1980) Antibiotic therapy of outpatient pelvic inflammatory disease (PID). Proceedings of the 20th ICCAC, New Orleans, Louisiana, abstract 671

56. Gjonnaess H, Dalaker K, Urnes A, et al. (1981) Treatment of pelvic inflammatory disease. Effects of lymecycline and clindamycin. Curr Therap Res 29: 885–892

57. Gjonnaess H (1979) Doxycycline in pelvic inflammatory disease. Curr Therap Res 26: 745–751

58. Mårdh PA, Moller BR, Ingerslev HJ, Nussler E, Westrom L, Wolner-Hannsen P (1981) Endometritis caused by *Chlamydia trachomatis* infection. Br J Vener Dis 57: 191

59. Gump DW, Dickstein S, Gibson M (1981) Endometritis related to *Chlamydia trachomatis* infection. Ann Intern Med 95: 61

60. Muller-Schoop JW, Wang SP, Munzinger J, et al. (1978) *Chlamydia trachomatis* as a possible cause of peritonitis and perihepatitis in young women. Br J Vener Dis 1: 1022

61. Hammerschlag MR, Chandler JW, Alexander ER, et al. (1980) Erythromycin ointment for ocular prophylaxis of neonatal chlamydial infection. JAMA 244: 2291–2293

62. Beem M, Saxon E, Tipple M (1977) *Chlamydia trachomatis* conjunctivitis in infants. Presented at the 17th ICCAC, New York, abstract 12

63. Beem MO, Saxon E, Tipple MA (1979) Treatment of chlamydial pneumonia of infancy. Pediatrics 63: 198–203

64. Rees E, Tait IA, Hobson D, et al. (1981) Persistence of chlamydial infection after treatment for neonatal conjuncitivis. Arch Dis Child 56: 193–198

65. Bell TA, Sandstrom IN, Fernarr KJ, et al. (to be published) Failure to eradicate infant *C. trachomatis* infection with a 10 day course of erythromycin.

66. Stamm WE, Guinan ME, Johnson C, et al. (1984) Effect of treatment regiments for *N. gonorrhoeae* on simultaneous infection with *C. trachomatis*, N Engl J Med 310: 545–549

Chlamydial Pelvic Inflammatory Disease

Per-Anders Mårdh

Institute of Clinical Bacteriology, University of Uppsala, Box 552, 751 22 Uppsala, Sweden

Introduction

During the last decade it has been established that *Chlamydia trachomatis* is a common, if not the most common, etiological agent of uncomplicated genital infections in the male (viz., of nongonococcal urethritis) and in the female (viz., of cervicitis) [1-4]. Since 1977 it has also been known that *C. trachomatis* can ascend to the upper genital tract and infect the epididymis [5] and the fallopian tubes [6].

The etiology of salpingitis has remained unclear. In earlier days, and still in certain geographic areas, specific infections such as tuberculosis and syphilis were common causes of salpingitis. In those days the etiology could often be confirmed histologically, since extirpation of the tubes (and the uterus) was often undertaken. In most industrialized countries the prevalence of genital tuberculosis has markedly decreased, particularly in areas where bovine tuberculosis has been eradicated [7, 8]. In cases of salpingitis in which a specific etiology could not be established, the designation "nonspecific" was used.

About one hundred years ago it became obvious that a proportion of cases of complicated nonspecific genital infections were caused by gonococcal infection. Some decades ago these infections seem often to have run a more severe course than is usually seen today; infections with septic manifestations and pelvic peritonitis and abscess formation were common. In these cases extirpation of the affected internal genital organs often had to be performed. Whether these manifestations could be ascribed entirely to the gonococcal infection or whether there was also a concomitant infection (or possibly superinfection) with other types of bacteria, e.g., with anaerobes and/or streptococci, is not known. In certain areas gonococcal and anaerobic infections are still common causative agents in pelvic inflammatory disease (PID); the latter in obstetric cases [8].

The relative proportion in which tuberculous, chlamydial, gonococcal, and anaerobic infections are diagnosed in PID cases is influenced by a large number of factors, such as the study area (epidemiological, cultural, and socioeconomic differences), the diagnostic method (if visual inspection of the tubes is not performed, a high proportion of false diagnoses must be expected [9]), the sampling and specimen transport methods used, the laboratory techniques employed, and awareness of the disease among the patients and the physicians in the study area (results of studies on patients consulting late in the course of the disease and with severe symptoms might differ from those of studies on patients attending early and presenting

Chlamydial Infections
Edited by P. Reeve
© Springer-Verlag Berlin Heidelberg 1987

only mild symptoms and minor signs). As indicated below, the proportion of cases of chlamydial salpingitis for example, is markedly influenced by the inclusion criteria used in the study.

The present review will concern chlamydial infection of the upper genital tract of the female. Clinical, pathophysiological (including microbiological) and therapeutic aspects will be considered.

Epidemiological Data

Table 1 gives some data from isolation studies of *C. trachomatis* in patients with PID [6, 10-24]. A direct comparison between the results obtained at different centers can not usually be made, for some of the reasons given above, among others.

Table 1. Isolation frequency of *Chlamydia trachomatis* from women with acute pelvic inflammatory disease

Authors [ref.]	No. of patients studied	No. (%) of Chla-mydia-positive patients
Bollerup et al. [10]	56	15 (27)
Eilard et al. [11]	22	6 (27)
Eschenbach et al. [12]	100	20 (20)
Gjønnaess et al. [13]	65	26 (40)
Henry-Suchet et al. [14]	16	6 (38)
Mårdh et al. [6]	63	19 (30)
Mårdh et al. [15]	60	23 (38)
Møller et al. [16]	166	37 (22)
Osser and Persson [17]	111	54 (47)
Paavonen et al. [18]	106	27 (26)
Paavonen [19]	228	69 (30)
Paavonen et al. [20]	101	32 (32)
Ripa et al. [21]	156	52 (33)
Sweet et al. [22]	26	2 (8)
Sweet et al. [23]	39	2 (5)
Thompson et al. [24]	30	3 (10)

Even studies from the same department involving different gynecologists (using different or even in principle the same sampling technique), particularity when performed at different times, can have different outcomes. For example, in Lund, Sweden, gonorrhea was diagnosed in every second PID case in the mid-1960s, while approximately only 10%-20% of such cases were diagnosed as being infected with gonococci 10-12 years later [47]. A number of more or less unexpected factors has be found to influence the culture results, such as the discovery that calcium-alginate-tipped sampling swabs – earlier generally recommended for sampling for chlamydiae – were toxic to the organism. When such a sampling swab was changed for one with plain cotton, the recovery of *C. trachomatis* from the cervix could be doubled [26]. When samples from the tubes are studied, the technique for collection of the samples is important to the outcome of culture studies. Thus a sampling stick with a conical cotton tip probably provides the best sampling tool by which the endotubes can be swabbed if the abdominal ostia are closed, puncture of the tubes and aspiration of the contents is preferable. Biopsy samples from the tubal fimbriae have been used for isolation purposes [27]. If laparotomy or laparoscopy is not performed, culdocentesis may be carried out to obtain samples for culture studies. However, such fluid seldom yields chlamydiae. The risk of contamination from the vagina and the intestinal tract cannot be overlooked. Recently, also, protected aspiration methods have been used to collect material from the uterine cavity [27]. A comparatively good selectivity can be achieved. It is notable that in some PID cases, chlamydiae can be isolated from the uterine cavity even though cervical cultures are negative for *C. trachomatis* [28]. In some such cases, chlamydiae have been isolated from the fallopian tubes. In some patients with salpingitis, *C. trachomatis* can also be recovered from the liver surface. In the case of endometrial, tubal, and perihepatic samples, the sensitivity of the culture technique used is probably of more importance for the isolation of chlamydiae than in the case of cervical samples, since fewer organisms are usually present in the latter types of samples. Chlamydial antibodies in cervical, but not in endometrial and tubal samples, might explain the discrepancy in certain patients between the results of cultures from these sites and the cervix. Among isolation techniques using McCoy cells, the method using cycloheximide [30], which we developed in Lund in 1977, has been found in experimental studies to be the most sensitive [31].

The use of monoclonal antibodies in immunofluorescence tests as well as ELIZA methods, has raised new possibilities for the detection of antigen *(C. trachomatis)* directly in clinical samples [32].

Serological Studies

The results of some studies seeking antibodies to *C. trachomatis* in patients with salpingitis are shown in Table 2 [6, 12, 15–21, 23, 33]. There are a number of problems with the serological diagnosis of chlamydial infections in acute salpingitis. Many of the patients with this disease have had one or more previous episodes of exposure to *C. trachomatis* – often with different immunotypes. Thus a primary immune response with formation of IgM antibodies can often not be expected. The salpingitis patient has often had cervicitis or in some cases cervicitis/endometritis for some time before developing salpingitis, so that a significant antibody response cannot be detected; from an immunological point of view the patient is already in the convalescent phase when attending. This is also true of the many patients who do not consult until many weeks have passed after the onset of symptoms [34].

Many patients with chlamydial salpingitis develop very high antibody titers [of microimmunofluorescent (MIF) antibodies] not commonly found in uncomplicated genital infections. However, some patients do not develop particularily high titers, or have stationary titers despite samples from the tubes being culture-positive. This makes it difficult to differentiate salpingitis patients from those with only cervi-

Table 2. Significant change in titer of microimmunofluorescent antibodies to *Chlamydia trachomatis* in women with acute pelvic inflammatory disease

Authors [ref.]	No. of patients studied	No. (%) with significant change of titer
Eschenbach et al. [12]	74	15 (20)
Gjønnaess et al. [13]	52	24 (46)
Henry-Suchet et al. [33]	27	15 (56)
Mårdh et al. [6]	60	22 (37)
Møller et al. [16]	166	34 (20)
Osser and Persson [17]	37	37 (51)
Paavonen et al. [18]	72	19 (26)
Paavonen et al. [19]	167	32 (19)
Paavonen et al. [20]	101	18 (18)
Ripa et al. [21]	80	28 (35)
Sweet et al. [23]	22	5 (23)

cal chlamydial infection on the mere basis of serological studies. In serological studies of series of nonlaparotomized or nonlaparoscopized cases with signs and symptoms generally associated with salpingitis, a proportion of cases of cervicitis are likely to be included. Thus, if the tubes are not visually inspected, cases of acute cervicitis can be misdiagnosed as cases of salpingitis [9].

To conclude, there are cases of salpingitis culture-positive from *C. trachomatis* from the fallopian tubes with a significant IgM and/or IgG antibody response, but there are also such cases with stationary antibody titers.

Cellular Immune Response

A cellular immune response to *C. trachomatis,* using TRIC and LGV antigens, has been shown in patients with salpingitis and culture-proven tubal chlamydial infection [35]. In leukocyte stimulation tests using the above-mentioned antigens, a significantly higher uptake of tritium-labelled thymidine was found in patients than in controls. No significant difference between chlamydial salpingitis cases with and without perihepatitis (see below) was found with regard to the cellular immune response to *C. trachomatis.*

Pathological Changes in Chlamydial Salpingitis

Chlamydial salpingitis may be mild, moderately severe, or severe according to laparoscopic criteria; tubal alterations range from reddening and swelling of the tubes to pelvic peritonitis with abscess formation [34]. Often there is a discrepancy between marked macroscopic alterations of the tubes and mild clinical symptoms [34].

In patients with salpingitis who are culture-positive for *C. trachomatis* and who have a significant antibody response to the organism, histological studies have been made on extirpated tubes [36]. The layers of the tubal wall, including the mucosa, the muscularis and the subserosa, are infiltrated by mononuclear cells and some polymorphonuclear leukocytes. The mucosa is totally or, in certain areas, patchily disturbed. There is an inflammatory exudate in the tubal lumen [36].

The fallopian tube seems to have a limited number of ways of responding to various infectious agents. Thus similar histological findings can be made in gonococcal, chlamydial, and anaerobic tubal infections.

In some chlamydial salpingitis cases, there is also peritonitis, periappendicitis [45 a], and perihepatitis.

Experimental Infection in Grivet Monkeys

Grivet monkeys *(Cercopithecus aethiops)* infected with *C. trachomatis* can develop salpingitis [37]. Thus if the organism is injected into the cervical epithelium, the uterine cavity, or directly into the fallopian tubes, salpingitis occurs. In such monkeys endometritis, perihepatitis, and splenitis have also been demonstrated [37]. The pathological changes, both macroscopic and microscopic, are very similar to those occurring in naturally infected women. The grivet monkey is similar to women with regard to the anatomy and in several respects to the physiology of the genital tract, making this monkey a very suitable experimental animal. If the tubes are occluded by a ligature (around the tubal isthmus) before chlamydiae are inoculated into the uterine cavity, salpingitis does not develop [38]. This indicates that a canalicular spread is the most likely route of infection in chlamydial salpingitis.

In primary infections of grivet monkeys a significant IgM antibody response has been demonstrated, where the antibodies were detectable in serum after 1–2 weeks and had disappeared after approximately 5 weeks. IgG antibodies appeared after 2 weeks and persisted at least for months [32]. Whether experimentally infected grivet monkeys also develop a cellular immune response to *C. trachomatis* is not known.

In grivet monkeys with experimental salpingitis caused by *C. trachomatis* which were subjected to repeated laparotomy and biopsy studies, it was found that the tubes may show narrowing of the lumina and mucosal occlusion during the course of the infection [38].

To sum up the experimental studies, it can be established that they have confirmed Kock's postulate that *C. trachomatis* is an etiological agent of acute salpingitis.

Clinical Characteristics of Chlamydial Salpingitis

The patient with chlamydial salpingitis is generally younger than the patient with salpingitis of other etiology. Three-quarters are under 25 years of age [25]. The chlamydia-infected patient has generally had abdominal pain for a longer period of time than other salpingitis patients and is less often febrile (i. e., having a rectal tem-

perature of 38 °C) on admission [34]. In conformity with the comparatively long period of time before consulting, the erythrocyte sedimentation rate is usually higher
than in women in whom the tubal infection is associated with other etiological
agents than *C. trachomatis*. As already mentioned, it is also notable that the laparoscopic findings are often more severe than might be expected from the relatively benign clinical course of chlamydial salpingitis [34].

No difference with regard to previous pregnancies, uncomplicated genital infections, PID and contraceptive method used was found between chlamydial salpingitis patients and patients with salpingitis of other etiologies [40].

Other Organs than the Tubes which May Be Affected in Chlamydial Salpingitis

A proportion of cases of salpingitis present with nonmenstrual vaginal bleeding, the
origin of which is the endometrium. Bleeding from the fallopian tubes in salpingitis
does not generally occur. Blood appearing in the abdominal ostia is rarely a feature
of this condition. Endometritis is a common finding in chlamydial salpingitis [28],
reflecting the canalicular spread of chlamydiae to the tubes. The chlamydial infection of the endometrium is characterized by a heavy plasma cell infiltration [41]. The
histological findings are similar to those described as characteristic of gonococcal
infection of the tubes.

Another rather common manifestation of chlamydial salpingitis is perihepatitis,
which is characterized by a fibrinous membrane on the liver surface with little inflammatory reaction in the liver parenchyma [13, 42, 44]. These patients may present
with sudden onset of sharp pain under the right arcus. The perihepatitis may also be
more or less symptomless and may be discovered accidentally at laparoscopy [42].
Chlamydiae may, as mentioned earlier, be isolated from the liver surface [29]. The
fact that *C. trachomatis* cannot regularly be isolated from the liver surface has raised
speculations as to whether an immunological reaction may be of importance in the
pathogenesis of perihepatitis.

Perihepatitis does not only occur after gonococcal and chlamydial salpingitis
but also in women with salpingitis in whom infection with neither of these organisms can be established [13]. It can also be demonstrated in women with peritonitis
without evidence of salpingitis [45]. The "violin string" adhesions considered typical
of gonococcal peritonitis do occur also in chlamydial perihepatitis. It should also be
remembered that such adhesions occur in patients previously subjected to abdominal surgery without evidence of genital infection.

In some patients with chlamydial salpingitis, periappendicitis has also been diagnosed [45 a]. Whether the periappendicitis is caused by spread of chlamydiae *per
continuitatem* from the fallopian tubes or whether other pathogenetic mechanisms
are involved is not known. In experimental infections with *C. trachomatis* in grivet
monkeys, splenitis has, as mentioned, been found in animals with signs of salpingitis [38]. Whether splenitis also occurs in naturally infected hosts is, however, not
known.

Estimation of the Risk of Developing Salpingitis For Women Harboring *Chlamydia trachomatis* in the Lower Genital Tract

We [46] have estimated the risk of women harboring *C. trachomatis* in the cervix and/or the urethra to develop acute salpingitis. In a defined population of approximately 14000 women of between 15 and 34 years of age, the annual risk of acquiring a genital chlamydial and gonococcal infection was found to be 47.6 and 12.1 per 1000 women respectively during the study period 1977–1980. We found the risk of developing salpingitis in women with lower genital tract infection with *C. trachomatis* and with *Neisseria gonorrhoeae* to be very similar: 8.0% and 8.6%, respectively [46]. However, these estimates are based on the presupposition that the two organisms are equally easy to identify. If this is not the care, the risk of developing salpingitis may be greater when cervical chlamydial infection is present, assuming that chlamydiae are more difficult to detect than gonococci.

Epidemiological Offensives to Reduce Salpingitis

Asymptomatic carriers are more common among those harboring *C. trachomatis* than those harboring *N. gonorrhoeae*. This stresses the need to perform contact tracing [47], among other things, in order to reduce the risk of female carriers of chlamydiae developing salpingitis.

The mean percentage of carriers of *C. trachomatis* among 373 female partners of males with genital chlamydial infection in seven different studies (from Scandinavia, United Kingdom, and United States) was 57%, with a range of 45%–68% [cf. 47]. These figures are generally lower than those found for *N. gonorrhoeae* in female partners of males with gonorrhea. Whether the contagiousness of *C. trachomatis* is lower than that of *N. gonorrhoeae* is not known. Whether the discrepancy only reflects a greater difficulty in recovering chlamydiae than gonococci remains to be determined. In Lund, we [47] found 84 (66%) of 127 female partners of men with *C. trachomatis* infection to be carriers of the same organism. Of the 84 women only 62 (49%) had any symptoms. *C. trachomatis* occurred in 52% of 114 male partners of 105 women infected with this organism. Of the partners, 59% were symptom-free. Female partners culture-positive for *C. trachomatis* often have difficulty in determining when they contracted their infection [47].

To reduce the risk of women developing acute salpingitis and its sequelae (see below), culture samples for *C. trachomatis* should ideally be taken from all women consulting with signs of genital infection; whether or not they complain of symptoms.

Contact tracing and partner treatment are important offensives in the attempt to reduce the risk of the women developing salpingitis. Otherwise, the risk of reinfection is high. There are also data [48] suggesting that a search not only for chlamydiae, but also for gonococci, should be made in partners of chlamydia-positive but gonococci-negative patients. Unexpected, undiagnosed cases of gonorrhea can be found by such a routine. This probably reflects the fact that a proportion of these men represent "the hard core" of persons with sexually transmitted diseases.

An early institution of therapy in cases of salpingitis will probably reduce the risk of complications following tubal infection. However, so far there are no reliable data supporting this assumption. In fact, there are studies [49] which may be interpreted in a very nihilistic way. The risk of becoming infertile after acute salpingitis did not differ, regardless of the antibiotic therapy used (drugs with known efficacy in vitro against the most important etiological agents of this condition [49]).

Sequelae of Chlamydial Salpingitis

So far, few data on sequelae of acute salpingitis organized with regard to etiological agents have been published. One exception is the finding that infertility seems to be less common after "gonococcal" than "nongonococcal" salpingitis [50], that is, in patients with salpingitis from whom gonococci were and were not recovered from the cervix. These patients were not studied for chlamydial infection. It is known that approximately every fourth patient with gonorrhea also has a genital chlamydial infection [51]. To enable reliable studies on sequelae of PID to be performed, a long follow-up period is necessary. Until recently, it has not been possible to perform such studies with regard to chlamydial salpingitis, due to the fact that the etiological involvement of *C. trachomatis* in this condition has only been recognized since the late 1970s.

We (unpublished data) have recently made preliminary estimates of the risk of women with salpingitis infected with *C. trachomatis,* but with no other etiological agent of this condition being diagnosed, becoming infertile. The study comprised cases diagnosed during the period 1976–1978. The risk was estimated at 12%–13%, which corresponds to the risk of women having had one episode of salpingitis becoming infertile, regardless of the etiology of the condition [50]. After two or more episodes of this disease, this percentage increases considerably, to approximately 35% and 75% respectively [50].

Whether and, if so, to what extent chlamydial PID is also associated with chronic abdominal pain has not yet been analyzed. The increased risk of ectopic pregnancy has been estimated to be sevenfold in PID materials not organized according to the etiology of the condition [52]. Recent studies suggest an etiological relationship between chlamydial infection and tubal damage promoting ectopic pregnancy [52a].

Studies by Henry-Suchet and associates in Paris have claimed the existence of cases of chronic salpingitis which are culture-positive for *C. trachomatis* from the abdominal cavity [33]. These findings have, however, not yet been confirmed by other groups.

Studies of groups of involuntarily childless women or couples have shown that a "positive" chlamydial serology occurs significantly more often than in control groups [53]. Such groups have comprised women operated upon because of tubal infertility [54], women with tubal infertility undergoing laparoscopy [55], and women consulting for infertility problems and therefore subjected to hysterosalpingography (HSG) [53, 56]. IgG antibodies to *C. trachomatis* occurred significantly more often and at higher titers in these cases with than in those without signs of sactosalpinz.

Multiple regression analysis of parameters such as parity, previous abortion and PID, use of contraceptives, presence of adnexal mass, cervical isolation of *Chlamydia* and gonococci, serum antibodies to these agents, and certain types of treatment showed that the presence of serum antibodies to *C. trachomatis* most significantly predicted the occurrence of tubal damage as indicated by HSG findings. Doxycycline-metronidazole had a negative predictive value, suggesting some effectiveness of this therapy in preventing tubal damage [53].

References

1. Oriel D (1982) Infections of male genital tract. In: Mårdh P-A, Holmes KK, Oriel DJ, Piot P, Schachter J (eds) Chlamydial infections. Elsevier Biomedical, Amsterdam, p 93
2. Johannisson G, Löwhagen G-B, Nilsson S (1982) *Chlamydia trachomatis* and urethritis in men. In: Mårdh P-A, Møller BR, Paavonen J (eds) *Chlamydia trachomatis* in genital and related infections. Almqvist and Wiksell International, Stockholm, p 87
3. Weström L, Mårdh P-A (1982) Genital chlamydial infections in the female. In: Mårdh P-A, Holmes KK, Oriel DJ, Piot P, Schachter J (eds) Chlamydial infections. Elsevier Biomedical, Amsterdam, p 121
4. Paavonen J, Vesterinen E (1982) *Chlamydia trachomatis* in cervicitis and urethritis in women. In: Mårdh P-A, Møller BR, Paavonen J (eds) *Chlamydia trachomatis* in genital and related infections. Almqvist and Wiksell International, Stockholm, p 45
5. Berger RE, Alexander ER, Harnisch JP, Paulsen CA, Monda GD, Ansell J, Holmes KK (1979) Etiology, manifestations and therapy of acute epididymitis; prospective study of fifty cases. J Urol 121: 750
6. Mårdh P-A, Ripa KT, Svensson L, Weström L (1977) *Chlamydia trachomatis* infection in patients with acute salpingitis. N Engl J Med 296: 1377
7. Falk V, Ludviksson K, Ågren G (1980) Genital tuberculosis in women. Am J Obstet Gynecol 138: 974
8. Mårdh P-A (1980) An overview of infectious agents of salpingitis, their biology, and recent advances in methods of detection. Am J Obstet Gynecol 138: 933
9. Jacobson L (1980) Differential diagnosis of acute pelvic inflammatory disease. Am J Obstet Gynecol 138: 1006
10. Bollerup AC, Kristensen GB, Mårdh P-A, Lind I (1982) Laboratory diagnosis of *Chlamydia trachomatis* infection in patients with acute salpingitis. In: Mårdh P-A, Holmes KK, Oriel DJ, Piot P, Schachter J (eds) Chlamydial infections. Elsevier Biomedical, Amsterdam, p 171
11. Eilard T, Brorsson J-E, Hamark B, Forssman L (1976) Isolation of *Chlamydia trachomatis* in acute salpingitis. Scand J Infect Dis Suppl 9: 82
12. Eschenbach DA (1980) Epidemiology and diagnosis of acute pelvic inflammatory disease. Obstet Gynecol Suppl 55: 142
13. Gjønnaess H, Dalaker K, Ånestad G, Mårdh P-A, Kvile G, Bergan T (1982) Pelvic inflammatory disease. Etiological studies with emphasis on chlamydial infection. Obstet Gynecol 59: 550
14. Henry-Suchet J, Catalan F, Loffredo V, Serfaty D, Siboulet A, Perol Y, Sanson MJ, Debache C, Pigeau F, Coppin R, de Brux J, Poynard T (1980) Microbiology of specimens obtained by laparoscopy from controls and from patients with pelvic inflammatory disease or infertility with tubal obstruction: *Chlamydia trachomatis* and *Ureaplasma urealyticum*. Am J Obstet Gynecol 138: 1022
15. Mårdh P-A, Lind I, Svensson L, Weström L, Møller B (1981) Antibodies to *Chlamydia trachomatis, Mycoplasma hominis* and *Neisseria gonorrhoeae* in sera from patients with acute salpingitis. Br J Vener Dis 57: 125
16. Møller BR, Mårdh P-A, Ahrons T, Nüssler E (1981) Infection with *Chlamydia trachomatis, Mycoplasma hominis* and *Neisseria gonorrhoeae* in patients with signs of acute pelvic inflammatory disease. Sex Transm Dis 8: 198

17. Ossler S, Persson K (1982) Epidemiologic and serodiagnostic aspects of chlamydial salpingitis. Obstet Gynecol 59: 206
18. Paavonen J, Saikku P, Vesterinen E, Aho K (1979) *Chlamydia trachomatis* in acute salpingitis. Br J Vener Dis 55: 203
19. Paavonen J (1980) *Chlamydia trachomatis* in acute salpingitis. Am J Obstet Gynecol 138: 957
20. Paavonen J, Valtonen VV, Kasper DL, Malmkamäki M, Mäkkelä PH (1981) Serological evidence for the role of *Bacteroides fragilis* and *Enterobacteriaceae* in the pathogenesis of acute pelvic inflammatory disease. Lancet 1: 293
21. Ripa KT, Svensson L, Treharne JD, Weström L, Mårdh P-A (1980) *Chlamydia trachomatis* infection in patients with laparoscopically verified acute salpingitis. Am J Obstet Gynecol 138: 960
22. Sweet RL, Mills J, Hadley KW, Blumenstock E, Schachter J, Robbie MO, Draper DL (1979) Use of laparoscopy to determine the microbiological etiology of acute salpingitis. Am J Obstet Gynecol 134: 68
23. Sweet RL, Draper DL, Schachter J, James J, Hadley WK, Brooks GF (1980) Microbiology and pathogenesis of acute salpingitis as determined by laparoscopy: what is the appropriate site to sample? Am J Obstet Gynecol 138: 985
24. Thompson SE, Hager WD, Wong K-H, Lopez B, Ramsey C, Allen SD, Stargel MD, Thornsberry C, Benigno BB, Thompson JD, Shulman JA (1980) The microbiology and therapy of acute pelvic inflammatory disease in hospitalized patients. Am J Obstet Gynecol 136: 179
25. Weström L (1980) Incidence, prevalence, and trends of acute pelvic inflammatory disease and its consequences in industrialized countries. Am J Obstet Gynecol 138: 880
26. Mårdh P-A, Zeeberg B (1981) The toxic effect of sampling swabs and transportation test tubes on the formation of intracytoplasmic inclusions of *Chlamydia trachomatis*. Br J Vener Dis 57: 268
27. Mårdh P-A, Weström L, Colleen S, Wølner-Hanssen P (1981) Sampling, specimen handling, and isolation techniques in the diagnosis of chlamydial and other genital infections. Sex Transm Dis 8: 280
28. Wølner-Hanssen P, Mårdh P-A, Møller BJ, Weström L (1982) Endometrial infection in women with chlamydial salpingitis. Sex Transm Dis 9: 84
29. Wølner-Hanssen P, Svensson L, Mårdh P-A (1982) Isolation of *Chlamydia trachomatis* from the liver capsule of a patient with Fitz-Hugh-Curtis syndrome. N Engl J Med 306: 113
30. Ripa KT, Mårdh P-A (1977) Cultivation of *Chlamydia trachomatis* in cycloheximide-treated McCoy cells. J Clin Microbiol 6: 328
31. Evans RT, Taylor-Robinson D (1979) Comparison of various McCoy cell treatment procedures used for detection of *Chlamydia trachomatis*. J Clin Microbiol 10: 198
32. Tam MR, Stephens RS, Kuo CC, Holmes KK, Stamm WE, Nowinski RC (1982) Use of monoclonal antibodies to *Chlamydia trachomatis* as immunodiagnostic reagents. In: Mårdh P-A, Holmes KK, Oriel DJ, Piot P, Schachter J (eds) Chlamydial infection. Elsevier Biomedical, Amsterdam, p 317
33. Henry-Suchet J, Catalan F, Paris X, Loffredo V (1982) Antibody titer to *Chlamydia trachomatis* in acute salpingitis and obstructive sterilities. In: Mårdh P-A, Holmes KK, Oriel DJ, Piot P, Schachter J (eds) Chlamydial infection. Elsevier Biomedical, Amsterdam, p 183
34. Svensson L, Weström L, Mårdh P-A (1981) Acute salpingitis with *Chlamydia trachomatis* isolated from the fallopian tubes – clinical, cultural and serological findings. Sex Transm Dis 8: 51
35. Hallberg T, Wølner-Hanssen P, Mårdh P-A (1985) Pelvic inflammatory disease impatients with *chlamydia trachomatis* infection: Cell-mediated immune response to chlamydial autogen. Genitourin Med 61: 247
36. Møller BR, Weström L, Ahrons S, Ripa KT, Henriksson H, Svensson L, von Mecklenburg C, Mårdh P-A (1979) *Chlamydia trachomatis* infection of the fallopian tubes. Histological findings in two patients. Br J Vener Dis 55: 422
37. Møller BR, Freundt EA, Mårdh P-A (1980) Experimental pelvic inflammatory disease provoked by *Chlamydia trachomatis* and *Mycoplasma hominis* in grivet monkeys. Am J Obstet Gynecol 138: 990
38. Møller BR, Mårdh P-A (1980) Experimental salpingitis in grivet monkeys by *Chlamydia trachomatis*. Modes of spread of infection to the fallopian tubes. Acta Pathol Microbiol Scand [B] 88: 107
39. Ripa KT, Møller BT, Mårdh P-A, Freundt EA, Melsen F (1979) Experimental acute salpingitis in grivet monkeys provoked by *Chlamydia trachomatis*. Acta Pathol Microbiol Scand [B] 87: 65

40. Svensson L, Weström L, Ripa KT, Mårdh P-A (1980) Differences in some clinical and laboratory parameters in acute salpingitis related to culture and serological findings. Am J Obstet Gynecol 138: 1017
41. Mårdh P-A, Wølner-Hanssen P, Møller BR, Weström L (1981) Endometritis in chlamydial salpingitis. Br J Vener Dis 57: 191
42. Wølner-Hanssen P, Weström L, Mårdh P-A (1980) Perihepatitis and chlamydial salpingitis. Lancet 1: 901
43. Dalaker K, Gjønnaess H, Kvile G, Urnes A, Ånestad G, Bergan T (1981) *Chlamydia trachomatis* as a cause of acute perihepatitis associated with pelvic inflammatory disease. Br J Vener Dis 57: 41
44. Wang S-P, Eschenbach D, Holmes KK, Wager G, Grayston JT (1980) *Chlamydia trachomatis* infection in Fitz-Hugh-Curtis syndrome. Am J Obstet Gynecol 138: 1034
45. Müller-Schoop JW, Wang S-P, Münzinger J, Schläpfer HU, Knoblauch M, Amman RW (1978) *Chlamydia trachomatis* as a possible cause of peritonitis and perihepatitis in young women. Br Med J 1: 1022
45 a) Mårdh P-A, Wølner-Hanssen P (1985) Chlamydial periappendicitis. Surg Gynecol Obstet 160: 304
46. Weström L, Svensson L, Wølner-Hanssen P, Mårdh P-A (1982) Chlamydial and gonococcal infections in a defined population of women. In: Mårdh P-A, Møller BR, Paavonen J (eds) *Chlamydia trachomatis* in genital and related infections. Almqvist and Wiksell International, Stockholm, p 157
47. Thelin I, Mårdh P-A (1982) Contact tracing in genital chlamydial infection. In: Mårdh P-A, Møller BR, Paavonen J (eds) *Chlamydia trachomatis* in genital and related infections. Almqvist and Wiksell International, Stockholm, p 163
48. Thelin I, Wennström A-M, Mårdh P-A (1980) Contact tracing in patients with genital chlamydial infection. Br J Vener Dis 56: 259
49. Weström L, Iosif S, Svensson L, Mårdh P-A (1979) Infertility after acute salpingitis: results of treatment with different antibiotics. Curr Ther Res Suppl 26: 752
50. Weström L (1975) Effect of acute pelvic inflammatory disease on fertility. Am J Obstet Gynecol 121: 707
51. Ripa KT, Mårdh P-A, Thelin I (1978) *Chlamydia trachomatis* urethritis in men attending a venereal disease clinic. A culture and therapeutic study. Acta Derm Venereol (Stockh) 58: 175
52. Weström L, Bengtsson L, Mårdh P-A (1981) Incidence, trends, and risks of ectopic pregnancy in population of women. Br Med J 282: 15
52 a). Svensson L, Mårdh P-A, Ahlgren M, Nordenshjold F (1985) Ectopic pregnancy and antibodies to *Chlamydia trachomatis*. Fertil Steril 44: 313
53. Paavonen J, Vesterinen E, Mårdh P-A (1982) Infertility as a sequela of chlamydial pelvic inflammatory disease. In: Mårdh P-A, Møller BR, Paavonen J (eds) *Chlamydia trachomatis* in genital and related infections. Almqvist and Wiksell International, Stockholm, p 73
54. Moore DE, Foy HH, Wang S-P, Kuo C-C, Spadoni LR (1980) Association of *Chlamydia trachomatis* with tubal infertility. Fertil Steril 34: 303
55. Henry-Suchet J, Catalan F, Loffredo V, Serfaty D, Siboulet A, Perol Y, Sanson MJ, Debache C, Pigeau F, Coppin R, de Brux J, Paynard T (1980) Étude microbiologique des prélèvements coelioscopiques dans les annexités et les sterilités tubaires. J Gynecol Obstet Biol Reprod (Paris) 9: 445
56. Punnonen R, Terho P, Nikkanen V, Meurman O (1979) Chlamydial serology in infertile women by immunofluorescence. Fertil Steril 31: 656

Chlamydia Trachomatis Infections and Pregnancy

Margaret R. Hammerschlag

Department of Pediatrics, Downstate Medical Center, 450 Clarkson Avenue, Brooklyn, N.Y.
11203, USA

Introduction

The occurrence of chlamydial infection during pregnancy is of added significance,
since it may affect the fetus and newborn infant as well as the woman herself. Although cervical infection with *Chlamydia trachomatis* may not be associated with
specific clinical signs in most women, ascending infection leading to salpingitis and
perihepatitis has been well described [1, 2]. *C. trachomatis* is also transmitted to the
infant during parturition, leading to the development of conjunctivitis and pneumonia [3–6].

Many questions concerning the potential sequelae of chlamydial infection during pregnancy remain, most notably the relationship to prematurity and perinatal
mortality.

Epidemiology

Prevalence of Chlamydial Infection in Pregnant Women

The highest rates of isolation of *C. trachomatis* from women have been found in
clinics for sexually transmitted diseases. Isolation rates as high as 37% have been
described [7]. However, the organism has also been isolated from 4.6% of female
college students attending a university gynecology clinic [8] and 8%–9% of women
attending general gynecology clinics [7]. During the past 5 years there have been
several studies of pregnant populations, mainly in Northern Europe and the United
States. Depending on the population examined, cervical infection with *C. tracho-*
matis has been found in 2%–30% of pregnant women attending prenatal clinics
(Table 1). The highest prevalence was found in an unselected population of American Indian women [8a]. In most studies, chlamydial infection was far more prevalent than gonococcal infection.

Chlamydial Infections
Edited by P. Reeve
© Springer-Verlag Berlin Heidelberg 1987

Table 1. Isolation of *Chlamydia trachomatis* from pregnant women

Investigator [ref]	Year	Location	%
Alexander et al. [9]	1977	Seattle	12.7
Schachter et al. [4]	1979	San Francisco	4.0
Frommell et al. [3]	1979	Denver	8.8
Hammerschlag et al. [5]	1979	Boston	2.0
Mårdh et al. [12]	1980	Sweden	8.7
Hammerschlag et al. [24]*	1980	Seattle	{ 21.5 10.0
Heggie et al. [6]	1981	Cleveland	18.0
Persson et al. [13]	1981	Sweden	2.4
Martin et al. [10]	1981	New Orleans	23.0
Harrison et al. [11]	1982	Tuscon	9.2
Thompson et al. [20]	1982	Atlanta	11.0
Hammerschlag, unpublished data	1982	Brooklyn	11.0
Harrison et al. [8 a]*	1983	New Mexico	{ 30.6 24.3

* 2 different populations were examined in this study

Factors That Influence Infection

The pregnant woman with chlamydial infection is most likely to be younger than uninfected women in the same population. Frommell et al. [3] found 53% of their chlamydia-positive women to be in the 15- to 19-year-old age range, as compared to 27% of uninfected women. Alexander et al. [9] found the mean age of their infected women to be 20.3 years as compared to 23.1 for noninfected women, which is very similar to the ages reported by Heggie et al. [6] (20.5 years vs 22.8 years). Martin et al. [10] and Harrison et al. [11] in the United States and Mårdh et al. [12] and Persson et al. [13] in Sweden have also reported the same inverse relationship with age. Mårdh et al. describe a gradual decrease in the rates of isolation with increasing age; 10% of pregnant women under 20 years of age were infected with *C. trachomatis,* whereas 8.7% of those aged 20–24 years and 4.2% of those over 24 years of age were infected.

Persson et al. [13] found the rates of isolation to range from 7.1% of those women under 19 years of age to 0.5% in women 30 years of age and older. The rates of chlamydial infection have also been found to be higher in primigravidas. This finding may be a reflection of age, assuming that older women have had more pregnancies.

Another factor that appears to influence the rate of isolation of *C. trachomatis* from pregnant women is marital status. Chlamydial infection is more frequent in unmarried than married women. Alexander et al. [9] describe 33% of the infected women in their study as married, as compared to 76% of the noninfected women. Frommell et al. [3] reported that 66% of the infected women were married, as compared to 86% of the culture-negative women. Marital status may be another indicator of sexual activity; McCormack et al. [8] found the isolation rates of *C. trachomatis* to be directly related to the number of sexual partners in female college students. The majority of studies in pregnant women have not provided information on the association of chlamydial infection with the number of sexual contacts. The studies of Heggie et al. [6] and Hammerschlag et al. [5] did not find any difference in the marital status of infected and noninfected women. This may be due in part to the populations studied, since the overall number of unmarried women in both studies (83% and 68%) was high. No data on marital status or sexual activity are given in the two studies from Sweden. In pregnant women in an inner city hospital, Martin et al. [10] describe the isolation rates of *C. trachomatis* as related to both more than two lifetime sex partners and unmarried marital status (68% vs 52% and 76% vs 59% respectively).

In studies conducted in the United States, race was also an important factor affecting the rates of isolation of *C. trachomatis* from pregnant women. In five of seven American studies, *C. trachomatis* was more frequently isolated from non-Caucasian women. Harrison et al. [11], Schachter et al. [4], Alexander et al. [9], and Frommell et al. [3] found isolation rates to be higher in black women. In the Tuscon study [11], the isolation rate was 26.7% in blacks as compared to 9.2% in whites and 5.7% in Hispanics. Schachter et al. and Frommell et al. found the isolation rate in black women to be 45% and 27% respectively.

Several studies have also described an association between the isolation of *C. trachomatis* and the presence of other venereal diseases, especially gonorrhea. Martin et al. [10] found that infected women were more likely to have trichomonads on Pap smear (33% vs 19%). Harrison et al. [11] found that 33% of chlamydia-positive women had a previous history of gonorrhea, as compared to 5% of chlamydia-negative women. Alexander et al. [9] found 9% of noninfected and 50% of infected pregnant women to have a history of gonorrhea. However, other studies [3, 5, 6] did not find any significant increase in the frequency of gonorrhea or other sexually transmitted infections in the women with chlamydial infection as compared to noninfected women. These findings may reflect basic differences in the populations that were examined. The latter studies were in large inner city municipal hospitals with large black populations, whereas the populations studied in San Francicso and Tuscon were in university medical centers with larger middle class populations. The relationship of marital status and race to the prevalence of chlamydial infection probably reflects socioeconomic differences especially relating to the prevalence of sexually transmitted pathogens in general.

The reasons why the rate of chlamydial infection among pregnant women appears to decrease with increasing age are not clear. Mårdh et al. [12] suggest that the comparatively lower rate of infection in the older women may imply that chlamydial genital infection is self-limited or that older women are less sexually active.

Neonatal Infection

Infants born to women with cervical chlamydial infection are at risk of developing chlamydial infection themselves. Acquisition appears to be vertical at the time of parturition. As shown in Table 2, the transmission rate from mother to infant has been found to be approximately 50%. If there has been cesarean section, transmission usually will not occur unless there has been prolonged delay following rupture of membranes. There is no evidence so far to suggest that horizontal transmission may occur after delivery. The preeminence of vertical transmission during delivery is reinforced by the observation that chlamydial infection rarely develops in infants born to women who have negative chlamydial cultures prior to delivery [3-6].

Table 2. Development of chlamydial infection in infants born vaginally to infected mothers

Investigator	Ref.	No. followed up	No. of infants who developed chlamydial infection (%)			
			Total	Conjunc-tivitis	Pneumonia	NP Infection
Schachter et al.	4	20	10 (50)	7 (35)	4 (20)	3 (15)
Frommell et al.	3	18	8 (44)	7 (39)	2 (11)	3 (17)
Hammerschlag et al.	5	6	4 (67)	2 (33)	1 (17)	1 (17)
Heggie et al.	6	95	27 (28)	20 (21)	3 (11)	3 (11)
Hammerschlag et al.	15	36	17 (47)	12 (33)	3 (8)	2 (6)

NP, nasopharyngeal

During passage through the birth canal, the infant may be inoculated at several anatomic sites, including the nasopharynx, conjunctivae, and gastrointestinal and genital tracts. As shown in Table 2, the approximate risk of developing conjunctivitis is 30%-40%, that of developing pneumonia 10%-20%, that of developing asymptomatic nasopharyngeal infection 20%. Schachter et al. [4] found 20% of the infants in their study to have rectal infection. In an earlier study [14], the same investigators isolated *C. trachomatis* from the vaginas of two of six female infants born to infected mothers. The rectal and vaginal infections were not associated with any clinical signs or disease. Overall, the nasopharnyx appears to be the most consistent site from which *C. trachomatis* may be isolated in infants. In one study [15], 78% of infants with documented chlamydial infection had *C. trachomatis* isolated from the nasopharynx. Since the infant may acquire the organism at one or several sites, chlamydial conjunctivitis may not necessarily precede the development of pneumonia, as the infant may only be infected in the respiratory tract. Not all infants who have nasopharyngeal infection will subsequently develop pneumonia. When we prospectively followed up 12 infants with isolated nasopharyngeal infection, only four (33%) developed pneumonia [15]. In the remaining infants, the nasopharyngeal infection was not associated with any symptoms or disease. The infection disappeared by 6 months of age without specific therapy. Heggie et al. [6] also reported that only three of 18 (12%) infants with nasopharyngeal infection developed pneumonia.

Depending on the rate of chlamydial infection among pregnant women, the incidence of chlamydial conjunctivitis may range from 10 to 70 cases per 1000 live births and the incidence of pneumonia may be 5-40 cases per 1000 live births.

Clinical Manifestations of Chlamydial Infection
During Pregnancy

Cervical infection with *C. trachomatis* in pregnant women appears frequently to be asymptomatic. Mårdh et al. [12] state that they were unable to establish the diagnosis by physical examination alone and that none of the chlamydia-positive pregnant or postpartum women they examined complained of symptoms. This has been the experience of most investigators. Heggie [6] specifically did not find any relationship between the presence of a vaginal discharge and isolation of *C. trachomatis* from the cervix.

Although cervical infection with *C. trachomatis* is frequently asymptomatic, ascending infection can occur. Thygeson and Stone [16] reported in 1942 that the postpartum morbidity, including postpartum fever and endometritis, was significantly higher in mothers of infants with inclusion conjunctivitis than in the general population seen at their hospital. In 1971, Mordhorst and Dawson [17] also found a high rate of pelvic inflammatory disease in mothers of infants with chlamydial conjunctivitis. Rees et al. [18] reported in 1977 that 5% of all mothers of infected infants developed postpartum infection including fever, infected lochia, and pelvic infection. Ten of those women were found to have positive cervical cultures for *C. trachomatis*. All these studies were retrospective and examined selected populations; thus it would be difficult to draw any definite conclusions about the relationship of antepartum chlamydial infection to postpartum morbidity from these data. Wager et al. [19] investigated the relationship of route of delivery and maternal infection with *C. trachomatis* to intrapartum fever, early postpartum fever, and late postpartum endometritis. A total of 391 women were enrolled during the second trimester. The authors found that among women who were delivered vaginally, antepartum chlamydial infection was associated with an increase in intrapartum fever and late postpartum endometritis. Of the 32 women with positive chlamydial cultures, 9% had intrapartum fever and 22% developed late postpartum endometritis as compared to 1% and 5% of 359 chlamydia-negative women. The overall rate of puerperal infectious morbidity was higher in the women with chlamydial infection (34% vs 14%). Forty-four percent of the women who underwent cesarean section developed some kind of infectious morbidity; this was not associated with antepartum chlamydial infection.

Although intrapartum fever in this study was attributed to amnionitis, this was a clinical diagnosis. The amnionic fluid was not examined for cells or microorganisms, including *C. trachomatis*. The diagnosis of endometritis was also clinical; chlamydial cultures were not obtained from the endometrium. Cultures were also not performed for other pathogens, such as genital mycoplasmas. Thompson et al. [20] obtained prepartum cultures for *M. hominis* in addition to *C. trachomatis*. The authors found that infection with *C. trachomatis* and/or *M. hominis* was associated with a higher incidence of chorioamnionitis, postpartum fever, and endometritis. Since infection with both organisms was common, it was not possible to define the relative risks for each. Harrison et al. [21] studied 1365 pregnant women at the University of Arizona in Tuscon. Cultures were obtained for *C. trachomatis*, *M. hominis*, and *Ureaplasma urealyticum*. The investigators found that postpartum fever was associated with cesarean section, premature rupture of membranes, and infection with *M. hominis,* but not with *C. trachomatis* or *Ureaplasma.*

As with nonpregnant women, serology is of little utility in the diagnosis of chlamydial infection during pregnancy [22, 23]. Attempts to make an accurate serological diagnosis of genital chlamydial infection in women are often unsuccessful because the onset of infection is unknown and, therefore, the demonstration of a rise in titer is not feasible. In the studies where serology was performed, the percentage of women with antibodies usually greatly exceeded the actual number with positive cultures. Persson et al. [13] found 50% of the women in his study to have chlamydial antibodies with titers $\geq 1:32$. The frequency of antibody was independent of age. In the 1979 study from Boston [5], serum antibody of titer $\geq 1:8$ was found in 73% of the pregnant women examined; antibody in cervical secretions was found in 47%. Hammerschlag et al. [24] in Seattle also found that 48% of the pregnant women studied had serum antibody to *C. trachomatis* (titer $\geq 1:8$). The methods used in all the aforementioned studies were variations of the microimmunofluorescence method [25].

Relationship of *C. trachomatis* to Perinatal Morbidity and Mortality

Genital pathogens, notably the genital mycoplasmas, have been implicated as causes of prematurity. Maternal infection with *U. urealyticum* has been associated with low birth weight [26], and histological evidence of chorioamnionitis has been described in the placentas of infants colonized with that organism [27].

The majority of the prospective studies of perinatal chlamydial infection have not dealt specifically with the relationship of *C. trachomatis* to perinatal morbidity and mortality. Frommell et al. [3] did not find any significant differences in gestational age and birth weight between the infants born to chlamydia-positive women and controls. Heggie et al. [6] did not find any statistically significant differences in the frequency of premature birth, stillbirth, neonatal death, premature rupture of membranes, or spontaneous abortion. There were also no differences in the mean birth weights and mean Apgar scores between infants born to infected and uninfected women. In the Denver study [3], the women were enrolled at less than 32 weeks gestation, but it was not specified how early, or how many women were enrolled at specific times. The patients in Cleveland were cultured at 8-12 or 35-37 weeks of gestation, but only 131 of 1327 (10%) had cultures obtained at both times.

The results of subsequent studies that have specifically addressed the question of the relationship of chlamydial infection to perinatal morbidity and mortality are not entirely consistent. Martin et al. [28] at the University of Washington found a tenfold increase in stillbirth or neonatal death among chlamydia-infected women as compared to uninfected controls matched for age, marital status, socioeconomic status, pregnancy order, and race. A total of 265 patients were enrolled in the study and 18 (6.7%) were found to be chlamydia-positive. The women were followed up from 19 weeks' gestation until delivery. Infection with *C. trachomatis* was also found to be associated with prematurity and low birth weight. No spontaneous abortions occurred among the chlamydia-positive women before 19 weeks of gestation.

Thompson et al. [20] in Atlanta examined 490 pregnant women who were enrolled during their first prenatal visit but before the third trimester. The overall rate of *Chlamydia* isolation was 16%, and that of *M. hominis* 55%. The incidence of poor pregnancy outcome, which included abortion, stillbirth, prematurity, and neonatal death, was 15.2% in women infected with *C. trachomatis* and/or *M. hominis,* as compared to 8.5% in women not infected with either organism, which was similar to the relationship of these organisms to maternal morbidity. Individually, neither *C. trachomatis* or *M. hominis* were strongly associated with poor pregnancy outcome.

Similar findings were reported by Harrison et al. from the University of Arizona [21], who examined infection with *U. urealyticum* in addition to *C. trachomatis* and *M. hominis.* A total of 1365 women were enrolled, the majority before 16 weeks of gestation. The isolation rate of *C. trachomatis* was 8.0%, that of *M. hominis* 23.5%, and that of *U. urealyticum* 72.3%. Since there were only 7 stillbirths in the whole group, this outcome could not be examined. The investigators did not find any relationship between the isolation of *C. trachomatis* and the genital mycoplasmas and the occurrence of prematurity or low birth weigth. However, a subset of mothers with recent chlamydial infection as evidenced by the presence of serum IgM antibody against *C. trachomatis* did have a higher proportion of premature deliveries (21).

Actual occurrence of ascending infection during pregnancy has not been demonstrated culturally or histopathologically. Infants of chlamydia-infected women who are delivered by cesarean section generally do not acquire chlamydial infection unless there has been premature rupture of membranes. There is one reported case of an infant delivered by cesarean section where the membranes were ruptured at delivery, who subsequently developed pneumonia at 1 month of age [29]. *C. trachomatis* was isolated from the nasopharynx. The mother's cultures 2 months postpartum was negative, but she had received antibiotics for postpartum fever and abdominal pain. The authors propose that the infection was acquired in utero. *C. trachomatis* readily infects primary human amnion cell cultures [30], but amnionic fluid has also been demonstrated to inhibit the growth of *C. trachomatis* in vitro [31].

In the only pathological study available, Knudsin et al. [32] found a positive correlation between the isolation of *U. urealyticum* or *M. hominis* from the chorionic surface of the placenta and perinatal morbidity (prematurity and perinatal death); *C. trachomatis* was not isolated from any of the placentas examined.

There are several reasons why the results of the above studies are not consistent. The women were enrolled at different times during gestation; some of the morbidity reported by Martin et al. was confined to the second trimester. Cultures were also not done for other microorganisms, which may be very important confounding variables. Although Harrison et al. [21] did not find any significant association between the isolation of *C. trachomatis, M. hominis* and *Ureaplasma* and perinatal morbidity, the isolation of any one was significantly correlated with the presence of either of the other two. Thus it would be very difficult to differentiate the potential adverse effect of maternal chlamydial infection from the potential effect of infection with *Ureaplasma* or *M. hominis.* The placentas and products of conception were also not examined.

The major clinical manifestations of neonatal chlamydial infection are conjunctivitis and pneumonia. Both infections appear to be limited to early infancy.

Conjunctivitis

C. trachomatis is the most prevalent identifiable infectious cause of neonatal conjunctivitis, accounting for 17%–48% of all cases [33, 33a]. The incubation period ranges from 5 ro 14 days after delivery, but onset may be earlier if there was premature rupture of membranes. Conjunctival cultures of infants born to mothers with genital chlamydial infection are rarely positive before 3 days of age, which may be a reflection of the initial infectious inoculum. Asymptomatic ocular infection also appears to be uncommon. *C. trachomatis* does not appear to have a significant role in conjunctivitis in older chilren [34].

The clinical presentation and course of chlamydial ophthalmia can be extremely variable and unfortunately nonspecific [33]. Affected infants may have only minimal erythema of the bulbar conjunctivae or may have the classic "sticky eye" presentation with copious mucopurulent discharge, chemosis, and pseudomembrane formation. Infection may be initially unilateral, but usually will involve both eyes. Contrary to the case in adults, follicles are not present in the neonate because the latter lack the lymphoid tissue. The course is usually self-limited with a number of infections resolving several weeks to months after onset without specific therapy. Appropriate antimicrobial therapy does result in the termination of conjunctival shedding and a shorter duration of the signs and symptoms of conjunctivitis. Persistent infection has been described and can lead to corneal scarring which resembles some of the changes seen in trachoma. Mordhorst et al. [35] described severe chlamydial eye infection similar to trachoma in 14 individuals in whom the disease began during infancy. In a study conducted by Chandler et al. [36], four of eight infants who had chlamydial conjunctivitis were found to have superior micropannus at 1 year of age. Corneal scarring after chlamydial conjunctivitis has been reported by other investigators [3, 17, 37–39], but the risk to the individual infant is not known. In a subsequent study which we conducted at the University of Washington [15], micropannus was not detected at 1 year of age in any of 15 infants who had chlamydial infection. Seven of these had culture-proven chlamydial conjunctivitis. The route of therapy may be responsible for the difference in the results, since all of these infants were treated promptly with systemic antibiotics, whereas infants in the other studies received only topical therapy.

Pneumonia

In 1975, Schachter et al. [40] described an infant in whom pneumonia developed following chlamydial conjunctivitis. Both parents had culture-documented chlamydial genital tract infections. *C. trachomatis* was the only pathogen isolated from the infant's upper airway. In 1977, Beem and Saxon [41] described a series of infants with a distinctive syndrome of pneumonia. Of 20 such infants, *C. trachomatis* was isolated from the nasopharyngeal or tracheal secretions of 18. The serotypes of the organisms that were isolated were common genital serotypes.

Infants with chlamydial pneumonia present with a history of cough and nasal congestion. Onset is usually at between 4 and 12 weeks of age. On physical examination of infant is tachypneic and rales are heard on auscultation of the chest;

wheezing is uncommon. There are no specific radiographic findings except hyperinflation. A review of chest films of 125 infants with chlamydial pneumonia found bilateral hyperinflation; diffuse infiltrates with a variety of radiographic patterns, including interstitial reticular nocular ones; atelectasis coalescence; and bronchopneumonia [43]. Labor consolidation and pleural effusions were not seen. Significant laboratory findings include peripheral eosinophilia (≥ 300 cells/cm^3) and elevated serum immunoglobulins (IgG ≥ 500 mg/100 ml, IgM ≥ 110 mg/100 ml).

Initially, Beem and Saxon termed this an "association", inasmuch as they could not recover the organism from the lung biopsies of two of the infants in their study [41]. Histopathological investigation revealed an interstitial pneumonia without unusual histological features. Subsequently, Frommell et al. [43] recovered *C. trachomatis* from lung tissue of an infant with the pneumonia syndrome; however, cytomegalovirus was also isolated. Arth et al. [44] have reported isolating *C. trachomatis* alone from lung biopsy tissue of another infant with pneumonia; no other organisms were isolated. Histological sections revealed pleural congestion; near total alveolar and partial bronchiolar mononuclear consolidation with occasional eosinophils; granular pneumocytes; and focal aggregations of neutrophils. There were also marked necrotic changes in bronchioles. Chlamydial pneumonitis has also been produced experimentally in infant baboons by inoculating the organism into the trachea [45]. The resultant pneumonia and the histopathology in these animals were similar to those of the previously described infants with chlamydial pneumonia.

Although viruses – usually cytomegalovirus, respiratory syncytial virus, rhinovirus, adenovirus, and enteroviruses – can also be isolated from the upper respiratory tract of infants with chlamydial pneumonia, available evidence does indicate that *C. trachomatis* is the central etiologic agent. Infants from whom both *C. trachomatis* and viruses were isolated have the same symptoms and clinical and laboratory findings as those from whom *C. trachomatis* was isolated alone.

The prevalence of pneumonia due to *C. trachomatis* as compared to that with other etiologies was estimated by Harrison et al. [46] in a subsequent study. *C. trachomatis* was isolated from nine (30%) of 30 infants under 6 months of age who had radiographic evidence of pneumonia. In comparison, the organism was only isolated from one of 28 infants without pneumonia who were admitted to the hospital during the same period. The control infants were matched for age, sex, race, and maternal marital status. The study was conducted over a 9-month period. This relatively high prevalence suggested that *C. trachomatis* may be responsible for many pneumonias in infants hithertho considered to be viral in etiology. The clinical and laboratory findings in these infants were very similar to those found by Beem and Saxon [41]. In addition, the presence of serum antibody to *C. trachomatis* in a titer $\geq 1:32$ as determined by the microimmunofluorescence method and antibody in tears and nasopharyngeal secretions strongly correlated with positive cultures. A lung biopsy was performed on one patient and demonstrated a profound interstitial infiltrate of lymphocytes, plasma cells, and eosinophils. Moderate fibrous tissue proliferation accounted for some alveolar wall and peribronchiolar thickening. Cases of chlamydial pneumonia in infants have now been reported from Israel [47], Canada [48], and Northern Europe [49, 50].

There are few data on the long-term sequelae of chlamydial pneumonia. The histopathology suggests that there may be some degree of scarring with compromise of pulmonary function. Hammerschlag et al. [15], in a longitudinal follow-up study from Seattle, did not find any excess of respiratory illness in infants with chlamydial infection followed up for 1 year. The data from the other prospective studies [3, 4] imply that after recovery from the acute infection most infants do not have further respiratory difficulties. Harrison et al. [51] reported the association of some chronic respiratory sequelae in infants with lower respiratory disease due to *C. trachomatis*. The diagnosis of chlamydial infection was made by a retrospective serological analysis of paired sera from 47 infants aged 6 months and over who were hospitalized with either pneumonia or bronchiolitis. Ten (21%) of these infants had elevated antichlamydial IgM titers ($\geq 1:32$) and were thought to have chlamydial infection. The sequelae noted included persistence, of cough and abnormal functional residual capacity seen at 3–5 years after illness. Since culture samples were taken from none of these infants their illnesses could have had other etiologies. Even infants with nasopharyngeal infection without pneumonia may have brisk antibody response [15].

Relationship of *C. trachomatis* Infections to Other Respiratory Disease

The relationship of *C. trachomatis* infections to other respiratory diseases in children is circumstantial. Secretory otitis media was described in approximately one-half of infants with chlamydial pneumonia in one series [52]. Tympanocentesis was performed in 11 of these infants and *C. trachomatis* was isolated from the middle ear fluid of three. However, both Schachter et al. [4] and Hammerschlag et al. [15] did not find a significantly higher incidence of acute otitis media in infants born to chlamydia-positive women than in control infants. Two studies attempted to find *C. trachomatis* in the middle ear fluids of children with chronic serous otitis media [53, 54]. The children ranged in age from 9 months to 11.9 years. *C. trachomatis* was not isolated from any ear fluid, although it was isolated from the nasopharynx of one 22-month-old [53]. These results would suggest that *C. trachomatis* does not play a frequent role in chronic serous otitis media in children over 1 year of age. The occurrence of serous otitis in infants with chlamydial pneumonia is probably secondary to eustachian tube dysfunction resulting from nasopharyngeal congestion. Since the middle ear is contiguous with the nasopharynx, one would not be surprised to isolate *C. trachomatis* from that site.

Prevention and Treatment

Although there is a substantial body of data concerning the treatment of chlamydial infection in men and nonpregnant women, there are only two studies that have evaluated treatment regimens during pregnancy. Treatment of the pregnant woman has two objectives: to eradicate the infection and to prevent transmission of the infection to the infant. Oral tetracycline, which is effective in treating female genital infection, is contraindicated during pregnancy. A preliminary study of erythromycin base at a dose of 250 mg four times a day for 14 days found it to be effective in eliminating *C. trachomatis* from the cervices of pregnant women in the third trimester [55]. No chlamydial infection developed in 17 infants delivered vaginally to women receiving this regimen. In comparison, 13 of 22 infants born to women who were not treated developed chlamydial infection at some site. No adverse effects were noted except that 5% of the women reported gastrointestinal disturbances.

Bell et al. [56] evaluated amoxicillin 500 mg three times a day for 10 days in a randomized double-blind trial. A total of nine women received amoxicillin and six received placebo. Sexual consorts were treated with doxycycline when possible. Although the mothers who received amoxicillin had a slightly lower rate of positive postpartum cultures three out of nine vs four out of six), the occurrance of disease in their infants was the same in both groups. The authors conclude that amoxicillin is ineffective in eliminating *C. trachomatis* from the cervix in pregnancy. However, Alexander and Harrison [55] compared amoxicillin (2 g/day for 14 days) to erythromycin (250 mg four times a day for 14 days) and found the two treatment regimens to be equally effective. Chlamydial infection developed in one infant born to one of 18 women who received erythromycin, but no chlamydial infection developed in any of the infants born to 18 women who received amoxicillin. Clearly, there is a need for further studies to confirm these findings.

Amoxicillin would be a very attractive alternative to erythromycin for several reasons besides better tolerance. Absorption of erythromycin is erratic during pregnancy and it may not treat concurrent gonorrhea or syphilis. Although erythromycin is recommended by the Centers for Disease Control (CDC) for the treatment of gonorrhea in pregnant women who are allergic to penicillin, its efficacy has not been established [57].

Unfortunately, the treatment of pregnant women with chlamydial infection requires the availability of facilities for screening and the opportunity to screen and treat the sexual contacts too. There are no programs for routine prenatal screening for *Chlamydia* in the United States as there is for gonorrhea. Prenatal treatment will not prevent later reinfection and the risk of transmission during future pregnancies. At this time no one would recommend treatment of all pregnant women without positive cultures.

A possible alternative approach is modification of current practices for neonatal ocular prophylaxis. Currently, in the United States, some form of ocular prophylaxis against gonorrhea is required by law, although 1% silver nitrate is specified by only one-half of the states. Prophylaxis with silver nitrate does not prevent the development of chlamydial conjunctivitis, as is demonstrated in the prospective studies of maternal and infant infection [3-6]. A preliminary study from Seattle [25] has suggested that erythromycin ophthalmic ointment was effective. Chlamydial conjunctivitis developed in 12 of 36 (33%) infants born to chlamydia-positive women who received silver nitrate, but in none of 24 infants who received erythromycin. However, the incidence of nasopharyngeal infection and subsequent pneumonia was not altered by erythromycin prophylaxis. The ointment was administered in the delivery room.

Tetracycline ophthalmic ointment is also recommended by the CDC as an alternative to silver nitrate for prophylaxis against gonococcal ophthalmia [57]. However, the limited data available now suggest that tetracycline ointment is not effective in preventing chlamydial conjunctivitis. Goscienski [58] reported in 1970 the occurrence of five cases of chlamydial ophthalmia during a 2-month period at the Parkland Memorial Hospital in Dallas. At that time 1% tetracycline ointment was used for ocular prophylaxis. Since no denominator was given, it is difficult to determine whether these cases represented individual failures or lack of efficacy. In a subsequent study from the same institution, examining the efficacy of intramuscular penicillin at birth for the prevention of group B streptococcal infection, tetracycline ophthalmic ointment was used as the control medication [59]. A total of 18 738 infants were enrolled over a 2-year period; 9439 received penicillin and 9299 received tetracycline ointment. During the study period there were no cases of gonococcal ophthalmia, but 22 infants who received penicillin and 18 who received tetracycline presented with chlamydial conjunctivitis. No culture samples were taken from the mothers before delivery and it is not known whether these cases are all that occurred. In an ongoing study in Tuscon, erythromycin ointment is being compared to tetracycline for prevention of chlamydial ophthalmia [55]. The preliminary results so far demonstrate equivalent degrees of breakthrough for both drugs, although the incidence of chlamydial conjunctivitis was less than was seen with silver nitrate. A potentially important difference between the Tuscon and Seattle studies is that in the latter, prophylaxis was administered when the child reached the nursery, not in the delivery room. Topical erythromycin and tetracycline are both relatively ineffective in treating established chlamydial conjunctivitis [60, 62]. The effectiveness of erythromycin as neonatal ocular prophylaxis may reflect antibiotic activity before complete absorption of *C. trachomatis* into the conjunctival epithelial cells: thus the timing of administration may be very important.

In the absence of adequate facilities for prenatal screening and treatment of pregnant women with chlamydial infection, neonatal ocular prophylaxis may provide a safe, cost-effective way of reducing some of the morbidity associated with neonatal chlamydial infection.

Treatment of Chlamydial Conjunctivitis

Topical sulfonamides have been the traditional treatment for neonatal inclusion conjunctivitis. Several studies have now demonstrated that any type of topical therapy is often inadequate. In a study initiated in Seattle [15] and continued in Tuscon [55], oral erythromycin, 50 mg/kg per day for 14 days, was compared to topical sulfonamide, also administered for 14 days, in the treatment of chlamydial conjunctivitis. Only seven of 18 (39%) of the infants who received the topical sulfonamide were culture negative and asymptomatic after therapy, as compared to 13 of 15 (87%) of the infants who were treated with erythromycin. Furthermore, there was no persistence of nasopharyngeal infection in the infants treated with erythromycin, which was not true for topical sulfonamide. Similar results were also reported by Patamasucon et al. [63], who compared oral erythromycin to topical erythromycin ointment. Both preparations were effective in eliminating conjunctival infection in 80% of infants, but the erythromycin ointment did not eliminate nasopharyngeal infection. The lack of efficacy of sulfonamide drops may be secondary to lack of compliance inasmuch as instilling these drops in the proper dosage for 2-3 weeks may be difficult even for the most conscientious parent. Since chlamydial infection in infants involves multiple sites; and over 50% of infants with conjunctivitis will have concurrent nasopharyngeal infection, systemtic therapy is indicated. When oral erythromycin is used, there is no need to use a topical preparation at the same time.

Treatment of Chlamydial Pneumonia

There are no controlled trials of treatment of chlamydial pneumonia in infants. At present either oral erythromycin or sulfisoxazole appears to be effective in eliminating nasopharyngeal infection in infants with chlamydial pneumonitis. Although the pneumonia may be self-limited in some infants and resolve without therapy, most investigators in the field do recommend treatment, as therapy does shorten the duration of the illness, especially if the infant has been ill for less than 1 week. Beem et al. [64] in an uncontrolled study found that the duration of symptoms in untreated chlamydial pneumonia ranged from 24 to 61 days, with an average of 43 days. Treatment with either erythromycin ethylsuccinate or sulfisoxazole eliminated nasopharyngeal shedding and shortened the duration of symptoms. By 1 week, 83% of treated infants showed symptomatic improvement. In most treated infants, resolution of X-ray findings was evident within 1 month of starting therapy. Persistence of nasopharyngeal infection was usually associated with continuing symptoms. The dosage of sulfisoxazole was 150 mg/kg per day and the dose of erythromycin was the same as that used in treating conjunctivitis. Bot drugs should be given for 2-3 weeks.

References

1. Mårdh P-A (1980) An overview of infectious agents of salpingitis, their biology and recent advances in methods of detection. Am J Obstet Gynecol 138: 933-951
2. Wolner-Hanssen P, Weström L, Mårdh P-A (1980) Perihepatitis and chlamydial salpingitis. Lancet 1: 901-903
3. Frommell GT, Rothenberg R, Wang S-P, et al. (1979) Chlamydial infection in mothers and their infants. J Pediatr 95: 28-32
4. Schachter J, Grossman M, Holt J, et al. (1979) Prospective study of chlamydial infection in neonates. Lancet 2: 378
5. Hammerschlag MR, Anderka M, Semine DZ, et al. (1979) Prospective study of maternal and infantile infection with *Chlamydia trachomatis*. Pediatrics 64: 142-147
6. Heggie AD, Lumicao G, Stuart LA, et al. (1981) *Chlamydia trachomatis* infection in mothers and infants. Am J Dis Child 135: 507-511
7. Taylor-Robinson D, Thomas BJ (1980) The role of *Chlamydia trachomatis* in genital-tract and associated diseases. J Clin Pathol 33: 205-233
8. McCormack WM, Alpert S, McComb DE, et al. (1979) Fifteen-month follow-up study of women infected with *Chlamydia trachomatis*. New Engl J Med 300: 123-125
8a. Harrison HR, Boyce WT, Haffner WHJ, et al. (1983) The prevalence of genital *Chlamydia trachomatis* and mycoplasmal infection during pregnancy in an American Indian population. Sex Transm Dis 10: 184-186
9. Alexander ER, Chandler J, Pheifer TA, et al. (1977) Prospective study of perinatal *Chlamydia trachomatis* infection. In: Hobson D, Holmes KK (eds) Nongonococcal urethritis and related infections. American Society for Microbiology, Washington DC, pp 148-152

10. Martin DH, Faro S, Pastorek G (1981) High prevalence of chlamydial infection in an inner city obstetrical population. 21st interscience conference on antimicrobial agents and chemotherapy (ICAAC), Chicago, 1981, abstract 515
11. Harrison HR, Alexander ER, Weinstein L, et al. (1982) Epidemiologic correlations of genital infections and outcomes in pregnancy. In: Mårdh P-A et al. (eds) Chlamydial infections. Elsevier Biomedical, Amsterdam, pp 159-162
12. Mårdh P-A, Helia I, Bobeck S, et al. (1980) Colihisation of pregnant and puerperal women and neonates with *Chlamydia trachomatis*. Br J Vener Dis 56: 96-100
13. Persson K, Ronnerstam R, Svanberg L, et al. (1981) Maternal and infantile infection with chlamydia in a Swedish population. Acta Paediatr Scand 70: 101-105
14. Schachter J, Grossman M, Holt J, et al. (1979) Infection with *Chlamydia trachomatis:* involvement of multiple anatomic sites in neonates. J Infect Dis 139: 232-233
15. Hammerschlag MR, Chandler JW, Alexander ER, et al. (1982) Longitudinal studies of chlamydial infections in the first year of life. Pediatr Infect Dis 1: 395-401.
16. Thygeson P, Stone W (1942) Epidemiology of inclusion conjunctivitis. Arch Ophthalmol 27: 91-122
17. Mordhorst CH, Dawson C (1971) Sequelae of neonatal inclusion conjunctivitis and associated disease in parents. Am J Ophthalmol 71: 861-867
18. Rees E, Tait IA, Hobson D, et al. (1977) Neonatal conjunctivitis caused by *Neisseria gonorrhoeae* and *Chlamydia trachomatis*. Br J Vener Dis 53: 173-179
19. Wager GP, Martin DH, Koutsky L, et al. (1980) Puerperal infectious morbidity: relationship of route of delivery and to antepartum *Chlamydia trachomatis* infection. Am J Obstet Gynecol 138: 1028-1033
20. Thompson S, Lopez B, Wong K-H, et al. (1982) A prospective study of chlamydia and mycoplasma infections during pregnancy: relation to pregnancy outcome and maternal morbidity. In: Mårdh P-A, et al. (eds) Chlamydial infections. Elsevier Biomedical, Amsterdam, pp 155-158
21. Harrison HR, Alexander ER, Weinstein L, et al. (1983) Cervical *Chlamydia trachomatis* and mycoplasmal infections in pregnancy. JAMA 250: 1721-1727
22. Schachter J, Cles L, Ray R, et al. (1979) Failure of serology in diagnosing chlamydial infections of the female genital tract. J Clin Microbiol 10: 647-649
23. Richmond SJ, Milne JD, Hilton AL, et al. (1980) Antibodies to *Chlamydia trachomatis* in cervicovaginal secretion. Sex Transm Dis 7: 11-15
24. Hammerschlag MR, Chandler JW, Alexander ER, et al. (1980) Erythromycin ointment for ocular prophylaxis of neonatal chlamydial infection. JAMA 244: 2291-2293
25. Wang SP, Grayston JT, Kuo CC, et al. (1977) Serodiagnosis of *Chlamydia trachomatis* infection with the micro-immunofluorescence test. In: Hobson D, Holmes KK (eds) Non-gonococcal urethritis and related infections. American Society for Microbiology, Washington DC, pp 237-248
26. Braun P, Lee Y-H, Klein JO, et al. (1971) Birth weight and genital mycoplasmas in pregnancy. N Engl J Med 284: 167-171
27. Shurin PA, Alpert S, Rosner B, et al. (1975) Chorioammionitis and colonization of the newborn infant with genital mycoplasmas. New Engl J Med 293: 5-8
28. Martin DH, Koutsky L, Eschenbach DA, et al. (1982) Prematurity and perinatal mortality in pregnancies complicated by maternal *Chlamydia trachomatis* infections. JAMA 247: 1585-1588
29. Givner LB, Rennels MB, Woodward CL, et al. (1981) *Chlamydia trachomatis* infection in infant delivered by cesarean section. Pediatrics 68: 420-421
30. Harrison RH, Riggin RT (1979) Infections of untreated primary human amnion monolayers with *Chlamydia trachomatis*. J Infect Dis 140: 968-971
31. Wolner-Hanssen P, Weström L, Mårdh P-A (1982) Influence of amnionic fluid on the formation of chlamydial inclusions in McCoy cell cultures. In: Mårdh P-A, et al. (eds) Chlamydial infections. Elsevier Biomedical, Amsterdam, pp 283-286
32. Knudsin RB, Driscoll SG, Pelletier PA (1981) *Ureaplasma urealyticum* incriminated in perinatal morbidity and mortality. Science 213: 474-476
33. Rowe DS, Aicardi EZ, Dawson CR, et al. (1979) Purulent ocular discharge in neonates: significance of *Chlamydia trachomatis*. Pediatrics 63: 628-632
33 a. Hammerschlag MR, Herrmann JE, Cox P, et al. (1985) Enzyme immunoassay for the diagnosis of neonatal chlamydial conjunctivitis. J Pediatr 107: 741-743.

34. Gigliotti F, Williams WT, Hayden FG, et al. (1981) Etiology of acute conjunctivitis in children. J Pediatr 98: 531–536
35. Mordhorst CH, Wang S-P, Grayston JT (1978) Childhood trachoma in a nonendemic area. Danish trachoma patients and their close contacts. 1963–1973. JAMA 239: 1765–1771
36. Chandler JW, Alexander ER, Pheiffer TA, et al. (1977) Ophthalmia neonatorum associated with maternal chlamydial infections. Tr Am Acad Ophth Otol 83: 302–308
37. Forster RK, Dawson CR, Schachter J (1970) Late follow-up of patients with neonatal inclusion conjunctivitis. Am J Ophthalmol 69: 467–472
38. Goscienski PJ, Sexton RR (1972) Follow-up studies in neonatal inclusion conjunctivitis. Am J Dis Child 124: 180–182
39. Markham RHC, Richmond SJ, Walshaw NWD, et al. (1977) Severe persistent inclusion conjunctivitis in a young child. Am J Ophthalmol 83: 414–416
40. Schachter J, Lum L, Gooding CA, et al. (1975) Pneumonitis following inclusion blennorhea. J Pediatr 87: 779–780
41. Beem MO, Saxon EM (1977) Respiratory-tract colonization and a distinctive pneumonia syndrome in infants infected with *Chlamydia trachomatis*. N Engl J Med 296: 306–310
42. Radkowski MA, Kranzler JK, Beem MO, et al. (1981) Chlamydia pneumonia in infants: radiography in 125 cases. AJR 137: 703–706
43. Frommell GT, Bruhn FW, Schwartzman JD (1977) Isolation of *Chlamydia trachomatis* from infant lung tissue. N Engl J Med 296: 1150–1152
44. Arth C, Von Schmidt B, Grossman M, et al. (1978) Chlamydial pneumonitis. J Pediatr 93: 447–449
45. Harrison HR, Alexander ER, Chiang W-T, et al. (1979) Experimental nasopharyngitis and pneumonia caused by *Chlamydia trachomatis* in infant baboons: histopathologic comparison with a case in a human infant. J Infect Dis 139: 141–146
46. Harrison HR, English MG, Lee CK, et al. (1978) *Chlamydia trachomatis* infant pneumonitis. Comparison with matched controls and other infant pneumonitis. N Engl J Jed 298: 702–708
47. Sagy M, Barzilay Z, Yahav J (1980) Severe neonatal chlamydial pneumonitis. Am J Dis Child 134: 89–91
48. Embil JA, Ozere RL, MacDonald SW (1978) *Chlamydia trachomatis* and pneumonia in infants: report of two cases. Can Med Assoc J 119: 1199–1204
49. Hallberg A, Mårdh P-A, Persson K, et al. (1979) Pneumonia associated with *Chlamydia trachomatis* infection in an infant. Acta Paediatr Scand 68: 765–767
50. Dunlop EM, Harris RJ, Darougar S, et al. (1980) Subclinical pneumonia due to serotypes D-K of *Chlamydia trachomatis*. Case reports of two infants. Br J Vener Dis 56: 337–340
51. Harrison HR, Taussig LM, Fulginiti VA (1982) *Chlamydia trachomatis* and chronic respiratory disease in childhood. Pediatr Infect Dis 1: 29–33
52. Tipple MA, Beem MO, Saxon EM (1979) Clinical characteristics of the afebrile pneumonia associated with *Chlamydia trachomatis* infection in infants less than 6 months of age. Pediatrics 63: 192–197
53. Hammerschlag MR, Hammerschlag PE, Alexander ER (1980) The role of *Chlamydia trachomatis* in middle ear effusions in children. Pediatrics 66: 615–617
54. Jones RB, Kleiman MB, Tubergen LB, et al. (1980) Failure to demonstrate a major etiologic role for *Chlamydia trachomatis* in persistent serous otitis media: 20th ICAAC, New Orleans, abstract 525
54a. Schaefer C, Harrison HR, Boyce WT, et al. (1985) Illnesses in infants born to women with *Chlamydia trachomatis* infection: a prospective study. Am J Dis Child 139: 127–133
55. Alexander ER, Harrison HR (1983) Role of *Chlamydia trachomatis* in perinatal infection. Rev Infect Dis 5: 713–719
56. Bell TA, Sandstrom IK, Eschenbach DA, et al. (1982) Treatment of *Chlamydia trachomatis* in pregnancy with amoxicillin. In: Mårdh P-A, et al. (eds) Chlamydial infections. Elsevier Biomedical, Amsterdam, pp 221–224
57. Centers for Disease Control (1979) Gonorrhea. CDC recommended treatment schedules, 1979. Sex Transm Dis 6: 89–92
58. Goscienski PJ (1970) Inclusion conjunctivitis in the newborn infant. J Pediatr 77: 19–26
59. Siegal JD, McCracken GH, Threlkeld N, et al. (1980) Single-dose penicillin prophylaxis against neonatal group B streptococcal infections. A controlled trial in 18 738 newborn infants. N Engl J Med 303: 769–775

60. Rees E, Tait AI, Hobson D, et al. (1981) Persistence of chlamydial infection after treatment for neonatal conjunctivitis. Arch Dis Child 56: 193–198
61. Bell TA, Sandstrom KI, Ingham K, et al. (1984) Erythromycin vs. silver nitrate eye prophylaxis for chlamydial conjunctivitis and extraocular infection. Abstracts of the international conjoint STD meeting, Montreal, 17–21 June 1984, abstract 138
62. Beem M, Saxon E, Tipple M (1980) Treatment of *Chlamydia trachomatis* conjunctivitis in infants. 18th ICAAC, Atlanta, abstract 528
62a. Heggie AD, Jaffe AC, Stuart LA, et al. (1985) Topical sulfacetamide vs oral erythromycin for neonatal chlamydial conjunctivitis. Am J Dis Child 131: 564–566
63. Patamasucon P, Rettig PJ, Faust K, et al. (1982) Oral versus topical erythromycin therapies for chlamydial conjunctivitis. Am J Dis Child 136: 817–821
64. Beem MO, Saxon E, Tipple MA (1979) Treatment of chlamydial pneumonia of infancy. Pediatrics 63: 198–203

Immunity

Julius Schachter

Chlamydia Laboratory, Department of Laboratory Medicine, San Francisco General Hospital, Building 30, Room 416, San Francisco, CA 94110, USA

Introduction

The literature on immunity to chlamydial infection is confusing and, at times, conflicting. It is clear that we know little about immunity to reinfection with *Chlamydia trachomatis* or *Chlamydia psittaci*. Abundant humoral, secretory, and cell-mediated immune (CMI) responses are readily demonstrable following chlamydial infection. The quantitative responses are often directly proportional to the degree of involvement during the infection, with systemic disease resulting in exalted responses above those seen with localized mucous membrane infection [21].

One of the reasons for conflicting data in the literature is the multiplicity of systems that have been studied in efforts to demonstrate factors involved in immunity to chlamydial infection. There are no convenient animal models for human infection with *C. trachomatis* and this has had a limiting effect on studies on immunity to these infections [3]. Studies on the basic biology of the organism have identified a number of virulence factors (specific attachment to host cells, parasite-specified endocytosis, and inhibition of phagolysosomal fusion), but no virulence antigens have yet been isolated. Their existence is deduced because specific antibody inhibits those virulence factors [22].

Observations in Humans

There is considerable circumstantial evidence to indicate that resistance to reinfection following a primary infection, or exposure to chlamydial antigens, does exist. Some of the data supporting the potential for immunization are derived from the natural history of chlamydial infection. Relative resistance to reinfection appears to develop over time (for example in trachoma). In some trachoma vaccine trials that were performed in the 1960s, a short-lived protective effect could be shown (Table 1; reviewed in [24]).

Secretory antibody in tears (actually, presumably IgG antichlamydial antibody in tears) collected from trachomatous individuals has been shown to have a neutralizing effect in reducing infectivity of chlamydial inoculum for subhuman primates [2]. Complement-fixing antibody, which appears to be directed against the genus-

Chlamydial Infections
Edited by P. Reeve
© Springer-Verlag Berlin Heidelberg 1987

Table 1. Field trial of trachoma – PEB vaccine in Taiwan [8]

	% Trachoma conversion		
	1 yr	2 yrs	3 yrs
Vaccine	10	16	49
Placebo	4	8	47
Effectiveness	66%	47%	–

specific LPS, is not protective. It is unlikely that any antibody alone is sufficient to protect against chlamydial infection. For example, the newborn exposed to *Chlamydia* during passage through an infected birth canal is born with IgG antibody levels at equivalent titers to those seen in the mother. These infants are not protected against infection, as 60%–70% will seroconvert and approximately 50% can be shown to be infected by recovery of the organism [25]. Thus IgG antibody alone does not protect against *C. trachomatis* infection.

Evidence for resistance to genital tract infection is less clear, although age-specific infection rates do suggest that repeated exposure may have some protective effect (this is potentially confounded by age-specific behavioral and exposure differences). One study performed on men attending a venereal disease clinic in California had an atypically low infection rate for *Chlamydia* among men with gonorrhea [23]. Typically, 20% of men with gonococcal infection have concomitant chlamydial infection, but in this particular study only 5% of the men with gonorrhea were found to yield chlamydial isolates. Serologic studies performed in that population showed that 93% of the men with gonorrhea had antibodies to *C. trachomatis*, as compared to only 60% of men with nongonococcal urethritis (NGU). Only 5% of the men with gonorrhea had chlamydial infections, compared to 25% of the men with NGU. One possible explanation for this result was that the higher antibody levels reflected higher rates of prior exposure, which had rendered the men with gonorrhea relatively immune to the chlamydial infection. This speculation was supported by the observation that 20% of the women with gonorrhea who had been named as contacts of the men had chlamydial infections. Thus these men with gonorrhea had a relatively high rate of exposure to *Chlamydia* but had not become infected.

It has been shown that antibodies of the IgG, IgA, and IgM class do appear following a *C. trachomatis* infection and that secretory antibody can be found at involved sites [29]. Abundant CMI responses can also be demonstrated [5]. While it is clear that individuals with antibody are more likely to be infected than those without, indicating that the mere presence of antibody is not wholly protective, one study found that recovery of *C. trachomatis* from the cervix was inversely related to the titer of antichlamydial secretory sIgA [4]. This suggested that sIgA or another antibody may have been neutralizing the organism and perhaps had some regulatory effect on the quantity of agent being shed.

Animal Models

Subhuman Primates

Subhuman primates can be immunized with killed elementary bodies and serotype-specific resistance to reinfection can be shown on ocular challenge (Table 2; [9, 24]). Because resistance appears to be serotype specific, it is likely that the antibodies (if they are the determinants for immunity) are against outer membrane proteins and would be similar to the antibodies detected in the microimmunofluorescence test. It should be noted that the antigens responsible for inducing protection against trachoma infection in subhuman primates (and presumably for humans as well) are different from the antigens inducing hypersensitivity [11]. Hypersensitivity reactions appear to persist for longer periods of time than do protective responses.

Table 2. Pannus development in trachoma-infected monkeys [9]

First infection – no vaccine	0/313
Reinfection or vaccinated	58/1176 (4.9%)

The experiments by Taylor and colleagues aimed at developing a subhuman primate model for trachoma have shown that repeated infection is necessary to generate the pathological lesions typical of human trachoma in a subhuman primate model [28]. However, after recovery from a single infection the animals become relatively resistant to reinfection. Thus it would appear that the immune response takes time to develop and can be overcome by repeated inoculations within the "incubation period" of the immune response.

Male and female subhuman primates are susceptible to genital tract infection with human *C. trachomatis* isolates [3]. Primary infection appears to confer a modest degree of protection against homologous challenge. Duration of secondary infection appears to be shorter than that of the initial infection, particularly in those animals with higher antibody levels [10].

Lower Mammals

It is likely that some of the naturally occurring *C. psittaci* infections in mammals can be used, by inference, to generate information concerning human immunity to infection with *C. trachomatis*. Some of these models, such as the guinea pig inclusion conjunctivitis (GPIC) infection, have a series of features that are similar to naturally occurring *C. trachomatis* infection [14]. GPIC involves the eye and genital tract. It is sexually transmitted and can be spread by ocular discharges. Newborn guinea pigs can be infected at birth. GPIC infection seems to be restricted to epithelial cells. Initial ocular infection results in a relative immunity to challenge.

With GPIC, the best immunity has resulted from infection. Often infection at one site can induce resistance to reinfection at another site. The most dramatic example of this is where feeding the GPIC agent rendered animals resistant to ocular challenge [16]. These observations have been confirmed in the author's laboratory and suggest the priming of humoral immunity through gut infection and seeding of the conjunctiva with specific antichlamydial immunocytes.

The immunity is temporary (in that it wanes after about 90 days), is dose-dependent (it can be overcome with higher inoculum), and is not simply dependent on the presence of serum antibody [1]. In some studies the titers of circulating IgG antibody were found to correlate with immunity [12]. Elevated IgG antibody levels could represent a proxy for generalized immune status of the animal, as passive transfer of antibody is not protective [31]. Unfortunately, the conclusion is compromised because the antibody titers achieved by passive transfer did not reach the levels seen in previously infected animals. Some studies indicate that immunity is correlated with the development of local sIgA [15, 17].

Thus it appears in the GPIC model that the initial disease episode, which lasts approximately 3 weeks, resolves with the appearance of high titers of circulating and secretory antibody. Initial resolution does not appear to be dependent on specific CMI responses. It is clear, however, that the immune response is complicated, as infected animals also develop early CMI responses and it is likely that both CMI and humoral factors do play a role in response to infection [30]. Cyclophosphamide immunosuppression at a dose that presumably interferes with B cell function more than it does with T cell function resulted in delays of sIgA production and of serum antibody production and in recovery from initial infection, but did not prevent ultimate recovery from conjunctivitis [13]. Rank and Barron showed that doses of cyclophosphamide which inhibit humoral immunity and leave CMI responses intact prevent GPIC genital infection from resolving [18].

In naturally occurring *C. psittaci* infections in lower mammals, there is some evidence of resistance to reinfection [27]. Cattle that have aborted following chlamydial infection have appeared to be protected against subsequent attacks. There are commercially available vaccines for prevention of feline pneumonitis in cats and enzootic abortion of ewes (EAE). At best, these vaccines are marginally protective. Infection with heat-sensitive mutants and their use in experimental live vaccines may have yielded somewhat better results in EAE [19].

Williams and colleagues have performed some of the most exhaustive dissections of the immune response using mouse pneumonitis infection in the nude mouse as a model. Early experiments showed that resistance to reinfection was T cell dependent and that a T-cell-dependent antibody response appeared predominant [33]. With subsequent studies it became apparent that cell-mediated immune responses also played a role in resistance to reinfection [32]. Thus the current state of investigations indicates that both humoral and CMI responses cooperate in producing immunity to a fatal lung infection.

Components of the Immune Response

It is possible that lymphocytes play a role in controlling *C. psittaci* infection. Certainly, the study by Shoenholz showed that mouse peritoneal macrophages could be destroyed by the 6BC strain of *C. psittaci* when infection was activated, but when similarly infected macrophages were cocultivated with lymphocytes from immune mice, chlamydial infection was inhibited. This effect could be abolished if antilymphocyte serum was added [26].

Lymphokines, probably specifically gamma-interferon, have also been shown to inhibit the growth of chlamydiae (*C. trachomatis* and *C. psittaci*) [6, 20].

It is likely that antibody can play some role in resistance to *C. trachomatis*. Antibodies against the major outer membrane protein can inhibit infectivity of *C. trachomatis* strains in cell culture [7]. This antibody appears to prevent an intracellular event (possibly reorganization from elementary body to reticulate body) and thus does not inhibit attachment and penetration.

References

1. Ahmad A, Dawson CR, Yoneda C, Togni B, Schachter J (1977) Resistance to reinfection with a chlamydial agent (guinea pig inclusion conjunctivitis agent). Invest Ophthalmol Vis Sci 16 [6]: 549–553
2. Barenfanger J, MacDonald AB (1974) The role of immunoglobulin in the neutralization of trachoma infectivity. J Immunol 113 [5]: 1607–1617
3. Barron AL (1982) Contributions of animal models to the study of human chlamydial infections. In: Mårdh P-A, Holmes KK, Oriel JD, Piot P, Schachter J (eds) Chlamydial infections. Elsevier Biomedical, Amsterdam, pp 357–366
4. Brunham RC, Kuo C-C, Cles L, Holmes KK (1983) Correlation of host immune response with quantitative recovery of *Chlamydia trachomatis* from the human endocervix. Infect Immun 39 [3]: 1491–1494
5. Brunham RC, Martin DH, Kuo C-C, Wang S-P, Stevens CE, Hubbard T, Holmes KK (1981) Cellular immune response during uncomplicated genital infection with *Chlamydia trachomatis* in humans. Infect Immun 34 [1]: 98–104
6. Byrne GI, Kreuger DA (1983) Lymphokine-mediated inhibition of *Chlamydia* replication in mouse fibroblasts is neutralized by anti-gamma interferon immunoglobulin. Infect Immun 42 [3]: 1152–1158
7. Caldwell HD, Perry LJ (1982) Neutralization of *Chlamydia trachomatis* infectivity with antibodies to the major outer membrane protein. Infect Immun 38 [2]: 745–754
8. Grayston JT (1971) Trachoma vaccine. In: International conference on the application of vaccines against viral, rickettsial, and bacterial diseases of man. Pan American Health Organization, Washington DC, pp 311–315
9. Grayston JT, Wang S-P (1975) New knowledge of chlamydiae and the diseases they cause. J Infect Dis 132: 87–105
10. Johnson AP, Hetherington CM, Osborn MF, Thomas BJ, Taylor-Robinson D (1980) Experimental infection of the marmoset genital tract with *Chlamydia trachomatis*. Br J Exp Pathol 61 [3]: 291
11. Kuo C-C, Wang S-P, Grayston JT (1971) Studies on delayed hypersensitivity with trachoma organisms. I. Induction of delayed hypersensitivity in guinea pigs and characterization of trachoma allergens. In: Nichols RL (ed) Trachoma and related disorders. Excerpta Medica, Amsterdam, pp 168–176
12. Malaty R, Dawson CR, Wong I, Lyon C, Schachter J (1981) Serum and tear antibodies to

Chlamydia after reinfection with guinea pig inclusion conjunctivitis agent. Invest Ophthalmol Vis Sci 21 [6]: 833–841

13. Modabber F, Bear SE, Cerny J (1976) The effect of cyclophosphamide on the recovery from a local chlamydial infection. Guinea-pig inclusion conjunctivitis (GPIC). Immunology 30: 929–933

14. Murray ES (1964) Guinea pig inclusion conjunctivitis virus. I. Isolation and identification as a member of the psittacosis-lymphogranuloma-trachoma group. J Infect Dis 114: 1–12

15. Murray ES, Charbonnet LT, MacDonald AB (1973) Immunity to chlamydial infections of the eye. 1. The role of circulatory and secretory antibodies in resistance to reinfection with guinea pig inclusion conjunctivitis. J Immunol 110: 1518

16. Nichols R, Murray E, Nisson P (1978) Use of enteric vaccines in protection against chlamydial infections of the genital tract and the eye of guinea pigs. J Infect Dis 138 [6]: 742

17. Pearce JH, Allan I, Ainsworth S (1981) In: Adhesion and microorganism pathogenicity. Ciba Foundation Symposium n. s. no. 80. Pitman Medical; Tunbridge Wells, pp 234–244

18. Rank RG, Barron AL (1983) Humoral immune response in acquired immunity to chlamydial genital infection of female guinea pigs. Infect Immun 39 [1]: 463–465

19. Rodolakis A, Bernard F (1984) Vaccination with temperature sensitive mutant of *Chlamydia psittaci* against enzootic abortion of ewes. Vet Rec 114 [8]: 193

20. Rothermel CD, Rubin BY, Murray HW (1983) Gamma interferon is the factor in lymphokine that activates human macrophages to inhibit intracellular *Chlamydia psittaci* replication. J Immunol 131 [5]: 2542–2544

21. Schachter J (1980) Chlamydiae. In: Rose NR, Friedman H (eds) Manual of clinical immunology, 2nd edn. American Society for Microbiology, Washington DC, pp 700–706

22. Schachter J, Caldwell HD (1980) Chlamydiae. Annu Rev Microbiol 34: 285–309

23. Schachter J, Cles LD, Ray RM, Hesse FE (1983) Is there immunity to chlamydial infections of the human genital tract? Sex Transm Dis 10 [3]: 123–125

24. Schachter J, Dawson CR (1978) Human chlamydial infections. PSG, Littleton, p 273

25. Schachter J, Grossman M (1981) Chlamydial infections. Annu Rev Med 32: 45–61

26. Schoenholz WK (1970) Studies on *Bedsonia* latency. II. Effect of immune lymphocytes and of rabbit-anti-lymphocyte globulin (RAMLG) on infected macrophages exposed to increased incubation temperature in vitro. Z Immunit Aller Klin Immun 139: 359–371

27. Storz J (1971) *Chlamydia* and *Chlamydia*-induced diseases. Thomas, Springfield

28. Taylor HR, Johnson SL, Prendergast RA, Schachter J, Dawson CR, Silverstein AM (1982) An animal model of trachoma. II. The importance of repeated infection. Invest Ophthalmol Vis Sci 23 [4]: 507–515

29. Wang S-P, Grayston JT (1974) Human serology in *Chlamydia trachomatis* infection with microimmunofluorescence. J Infect Dis 130: 388–397

30. Watson RR, MacDonald AB, Murray ES, Modabber FZ (1973) Immunity to chlamydial infections of the eye. 3. Presence and duration of delayed hypersensitivity to guinea pig inclusion conjunctivitis. J Immunol 111: 618

31. Watson RR, Mull D, MacDonald AB, Thompson SE, III, Bear SE (1973) Immunity to chlamydial infections of the eye. II. Studies of passively transferred serum antibody in resistance to infection with guinea pig inclusion conjunctivitis. Infect Immun 7 [4]: 597–599

32. Williams DM, Schachter J, Coalson JJ, Grubbs B (1984) Cellular immunity to the mouse pneumonitis agent. J Infect Dis 149 [4]: 630–639

33. Williams DM, Schachter J, Drutz DJ, Sumaya CV (1981) Pneumonia due to *Chlamydia trachomatis* in the immunocompromised (nude) mouse. J Infect Dis 143 [2]: 238–241

Chlamydia Trachomatis: Biology of the Agent

Gerald I. Byrne

Department of Medical Microbiology, University of Wisconsin-Madison, Medical School, Madison, WI 53706, USA

Introduction

The genus *Chlamydia* is composed of two species of morphologically and developmentally related prokaryotic microorganisms. The chlamydiae are obligate intracellular microbes capable of replication only within the confines of a membrane-bound vesicle (inclusion) in the cytoplasm of susceptible eukaryotic host cells.

The chlamydiae are taxonomically separated from other obligate intracellular bacteria of eukaryotes (the Rickettsiales), principally due to their distinctive mode of intracellular growth and development and their unique morphology and ultrastructure. The presence of genus-, species-, and type-specific antigens also distinguishes chlamydiae from other intracellular or free-living microbes. The order Chlamydiales comprises just one family, the Chlamydiaceae. The two currently recognized species are *C. trachomatis* and *C. psittaci*[1]; the *C. trachomatis* species will be officially subclassified into three distinct biovars [2] in the next edition of *Bergey's Manual of Determinative Bacteriology*.

Chlamydia psittaci is ubiquitously distributed in nature, whereas *C. trachomatis* is, with one exception (that being the agent of mouse pneumonitis), exclusively a pathogen of man [3]. The latter species has been subdivided by a variety of classification systems, the most frequently used being based on type-specific antigens identified by a microimmunofluorescence test developed by Wang and Grayston [4]. The technique is an indirect method, where known *C. trachomatis* serotypes fixed to glass slides in organized patterns are tested against sera or local secretions from infected individuals. The presence of anti-*C. trachomatis* immunoglobulin directed against a particular serotype is determined by adding fluorescein-conjugated anti-human immunoglobulin to the test slide. There are currently 15 recognized *C. trachomatis* serotypes (A, B, Ba, C-K, L_1-L_3). A degree of cross-reactivity exists between serotypes, and this antigenic relatedness forms the basis of the so-called B and C serogroups. The antigenic determinants responsible for conferring genus, species, group, and type specificity are discussed in more detail in a subsequent section of this chapter.

Evolutionary divergence has occurred between the two recognized chlamydial species. This is documented by the observation that although oculogenital and lymphogranuloma venereum (LGV) biovars of *C. trachomatis* share considerable DNA homology, *C. psittaci* shares almost no homologous sequences with any of the *C. trachomatis* serotypes.

Chlamydial Infections
Edited by P. Reeve
© Springer-Verlag Berlin Heidelberg 1987

The A-K serotypes are responsible for oculogenital and related infections, while the L$_1$-L$_3$ serotypes represent a distinct *C. trachomatis* biovar. The L$_1$-L$_3$ serotypes are responsible for a relatively uncommon venereally transmitted infection (LGV) characterized by an initial benign chancre at the site of transmission, followed by extensive inguinal and often femoral lymphatic involvement. Progressive spread of the disease can also occur [5]. The LGV biovar is distinctive not only because of the clinical manifestations of infection, but also because these serotypes readily adapt to growth in vertebrate tissue culture systems. The A-K serotypes are more fastidious organisms, and more elaborate cell culture manipulations are required for their propagation [6]. This is an important consideration, since the most reliable diagnostic tool currently available for documenting genital or neonatal chlamydial infections is growth and identification of the organisms in cell culture [5]. A variety of tissue culture systems have been favored at one time or another, but currently centrifuging clinical material onto cycloheximide-treated mouse fibroblasts (McCoy cells), incubating the infected cells for 2 or 3 days, staining them with iodine, Giemsa or fluorescent antibody, and observing typical chlamydial inclusions by light or fluorescent microscopy is the standard method. Figure 1 shows a typical *C. trachomatis* inclusion in McCoy cells prestained with rhodamine-conjugated normal rabbit serum, then stained with fluorescein-isothiocyanate-conjugated antichlamydial immunoglobulin. The cells were fixed and stained 1 day after infection.

Several excellent reviews have been published on the biology of chlamydiae within the past few years [8-10]. Much of the knowledge concerning fundamental aspects of chlamydial growth and the interactions of chlamydiae with host cells has

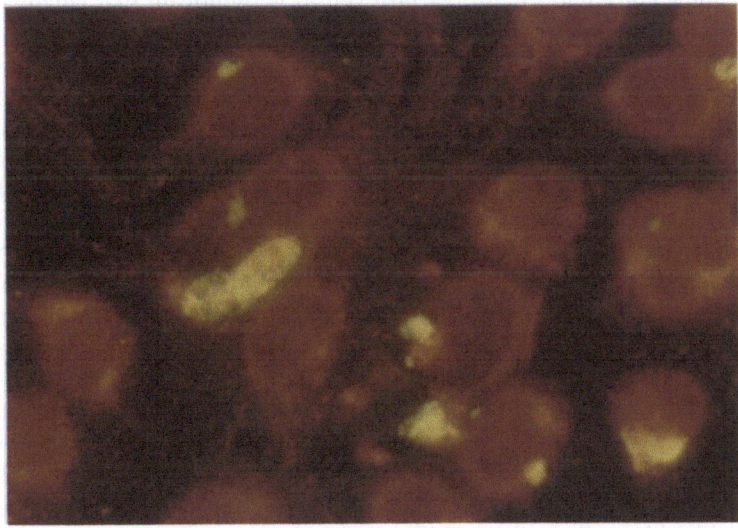

Fig. 1. *C. trachomatis*-infected McCoy cell stained with fluorescein-isothiocynate-conjugated antichlamydial antibody after being prestained with rhodamine-conjugated normal rabbit serum. Chlamydial inclusions appear as bright green cytoplasmic vesicles. The remainder of the host cell is stained rust orange. (Photomicrograph by courtesy of Dr. B. Z. Horvath) × 1000

been accomplished with laboratory strains of *C. psittaci*, since they lend themselves well to experimental cell culture systems and animal models of human infections. This chapter, however, is not intended to be an exhaustive review of the general literature, but rather a focused examination of new information specifically applicable to the biology of *C. trachomatis*. The description of the now classic cycle of intracellular chlamydial development will be directed with this point in mind, and special attention will be paid to how the unique properties of these intracellular pathogens may relate to the clinical manifestations of chlamydial infections, their diagnosis, and their control.

Host Cell Interactions and Metabolism

Interactions

The literature is replete with descriptions of the unique cycle of intracellular chlamydial replication [see, e. g., 5, 8–10 for reviews and bibliographies], termed the "developmental cycle". It is clear that certain criteria must be met in order for chlamydial growth to occur. Initially, they must somehow come in contact with, attach to, and be taken up by susceptible host cells. In the laboratory this process is facilitated by centrifugation of inocula onto cell culture monolayers specifically selected for their ability to support chlamydial replication [6]. In nature, however, chlamydiae must fend for themselves without the aid of mechanical devices, and judging from the prevalence of chlamydial infections in the world today, they have been fairly successful (that is, well adapted) at recognizing (in the molecular sense) and gaining entry into the proper host cell. It is significant that chlamydiae are under constant selective pressure for this particular fitness trait, so it should not be surprising that they have evolved mechanisms to help mediate the attachment and ingestion process. Oculogenital strains of *C. trachomatis* exhibit a tropism for the columnar epithelial cells of mucosal surfaces [5]. Implicit in the idea of tissue tropism is the concept of recognition and attachment specificity. Indeed, there is evidence that attachment of *C. trachomatis* occurs via sialic-acid-containing host cell binding sites [11], yet the specificity for this attachment must reside with the chlamydiae, since it is they and not the host cells that are under selective pressure to reach their particular habitat. The degree of hydrophobicity and the relative distribution of negative charges on the chlamydial surface may be essential to the attachment process. The former should be great and the latter small to promote the best initial contact [12]. The presence of heat-labile, protease-insensitive chlamydial surface receptors that recognize and attach to trypsin-sensitive host cell binding sites have also been demonstrated for selected strains [13], but these binding sites may very well not be present on A-K strains. In the laboratory [14] it is possible temporally to separate attachment from ingestion, but once they are attached the normal sequence is for viable chlamydiae to be rapidly taken up by susceptible host cells. The overall process resembles phagocytosis and requires expenditure of host cell energy (chlamydiae do not participate metabolically in this process), but is distinct from classic phagocytosis in that cytoskeletal elements are not involved [13, 15, 16] and lysosomes do not fuse with the resultant chlamydiae-containing endocytic vesicle [17]. Once uptake has been completed, chlamydiae remain within the membrane-bound cytoplasmic vesicle throughout their entire replicative cycle.

Soon after ingestion, a remarkable transformation occurs. For any given chlamydial strain, two distinct cell types exist. The cell that mediates attachment and uptake by host cells and has been the subject of the discussion thus far is referred to as the elementary body (EB). It is a metabolically inert cell, specifically adapted to the early events of host cell interactions and to the transitory extracellular existence encountered between hosts. EBs are small cocci, measuring only 0.2-0.3 μm in diameter (Fig. 2). Their external surface is composed of a rigid envelope that is characterized by the presence of hemispheric projections [18] organized into arrays of hexagons when viewed with the scanning electron microscope. Under the transmission electron microscope (Fig. 3), the outer envelope is seen as a trilaminar structure, and surrounds a trilaminar cytoplasmic membrane. The DNA is compacted into an electron-dense nucleoid, and few cytoplasmic ribosomes are observed. Shortly after EB uptake is completed, the small, sturdy EB differentiates into a larger coccoid form (Fig. 4). This larger cell is the replicative form of the organism and is called the reticulate body (RB). Reticulate bodies measure about 1 μm in diameter. They are extremely fragile when removed from the intracellular environment, and are incapable of initiating the infectious cycle. They metabolize, grow, and divide by binary fission within the inclusion vesicle. Septum formation is not thought of as

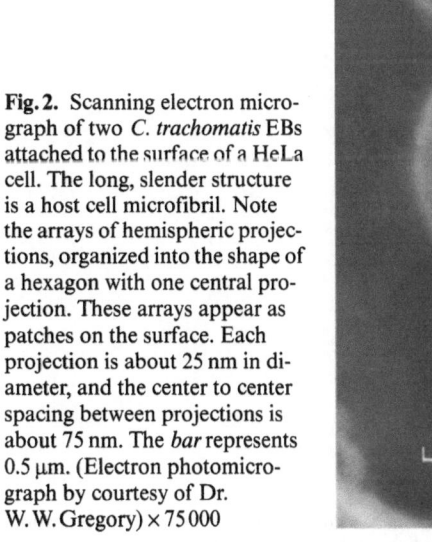

Fig. 2. Scanning electron micrograph of two *C. trachomatis* EBs attached to the surface of a HeLa cell. The long, slender structure is a host cell microfibril. Note the arrays of hemispheric projections, organized into the shape of a hexagon with one central projection. These arrays appear as patches on the surface. Each projection is about 25 nm in diameter, and the center to center spacing between projections is about 75 nm. The *bar* represents 0.5 μm. (Electron photomicrograph by courtesy of Dr. W. W. Gregory) × 75 000

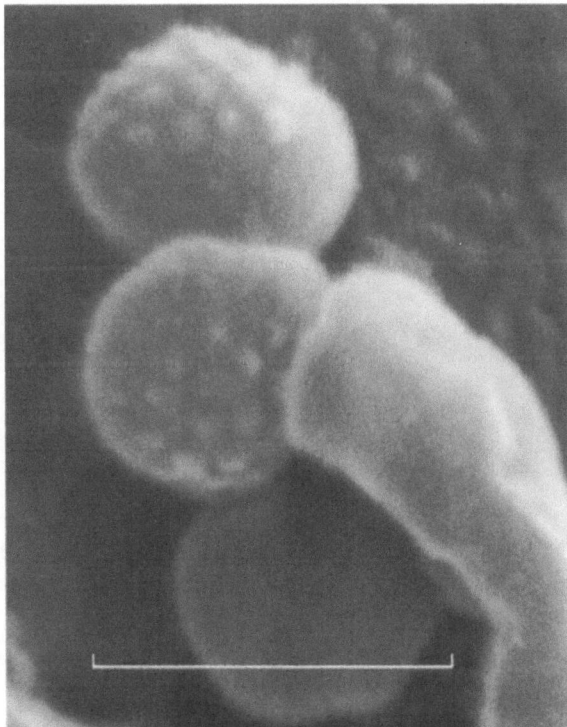

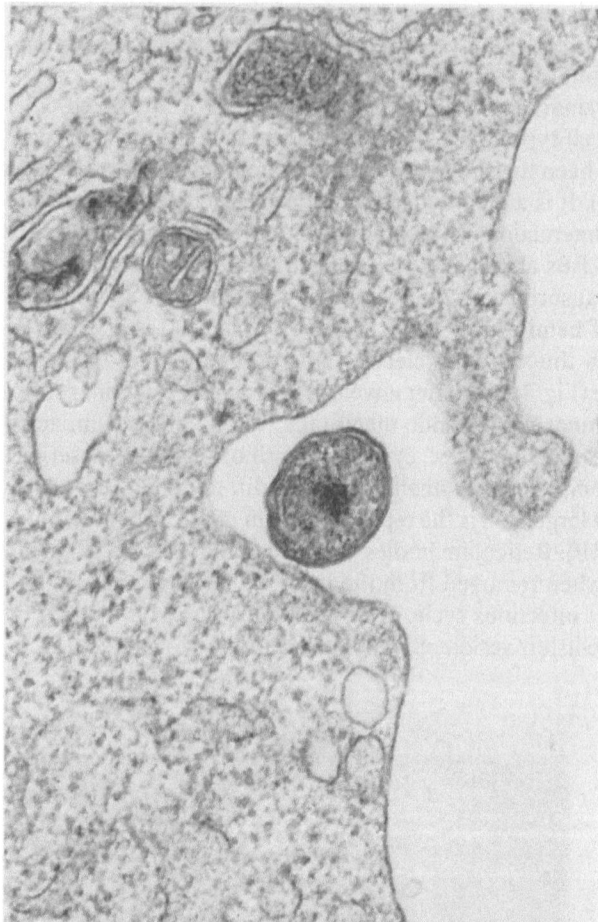

Fig. 3. Transmission electron micrograph of *C. trachomatis* EB attached to the surface of a HeLa cell in culture. Note densely packed nucleoid and double trilaminar envelope and membrane. (Electron photomicrograph by courtesy of Dr. C. D. Rothermel) × 27 000

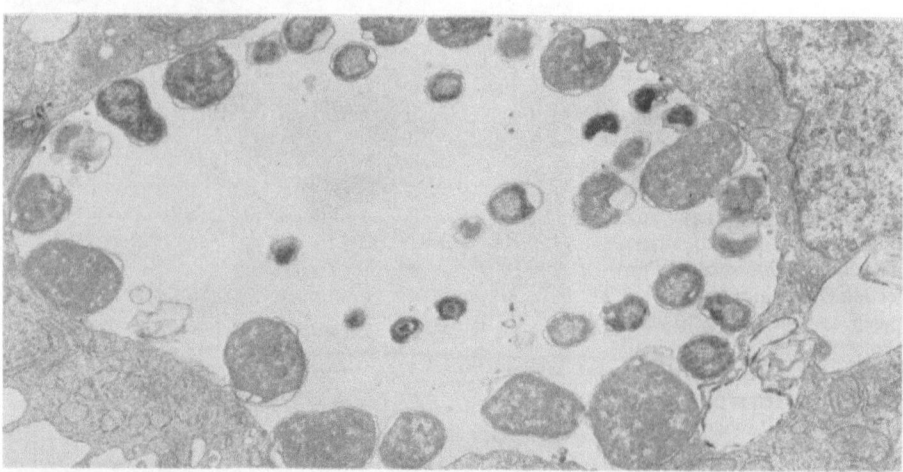

Fig. 4. Transmission electron micrograph of developing *C. trachomatis* inclusion. The inclusion membrane can be seen. Larger, replicating RBs are indicated. EBs may also be seen. (Electron photomicrograph by courtesy of Dr. C. D. Rothermel) × 14 000

part of this process, but occasionally septum-like structures have been observed in dividing cells (Fig. 5). No organized arrays of hemispheric projections are seen when RBs are viewed in the scanning electron microscope, yet RBs retain the tri-laminar outer envelope and cytoplasmic membrane morphology. Reticulate body DNA is not compacted into an electron-dense nucleoid, and cytoplasmic ribosomes are plentiful. Elementary and reticulate bodies each possess all species of RNA, but

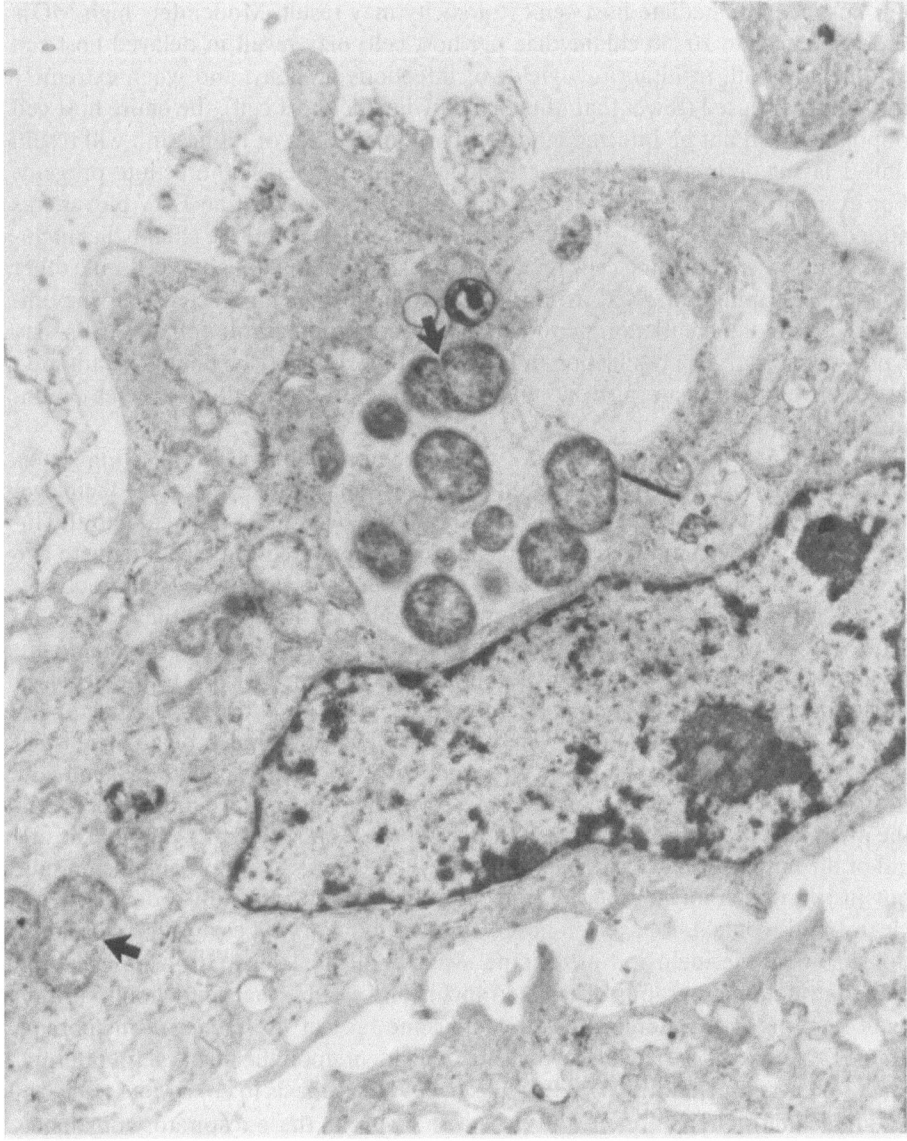

Fig. 5. Transmission electron micrograph of a *Chlamydia*-infected L cell. Replicating RBs are seen in two intracellular inclusions. Septa are indicated by *arrows*. × 10 000

during the transformation from EB to RB the RNA to DNA ratio increases from about 1:1 to about 3:1, a reflection of the heightened degree of metabolic activity present in the RB. Reticulate bodies continue to replicate within the inclusion vesicle for periods of time that are dependent upon the particular chlamydial strain, the host cell type, and in the laboratory, the type of medium and additives employed [see, e. g., 19–23 for various conditions of cell culture and their effects on chlamydial development]. The successful productive infection is dependent not only on the proper nutritional requirements and host cell type, but also on the multiplicity of infection (MOI). When the MOI is too high (i. e., greater than 100 or so chlamydiae per host cell), immediate host cell cytotoxicity may result. Moderately high MOIs (i. e., greater than 20–50 chlamydiae per host cell) may result in delayed host cell cytotoxicity, with resultant low yields of infectious progeny, and when extremely low MOIs are used (fewer than three chlamydiae per host cell), the entire host cell population will not be infected, and asynchronous cycles of replication will result, thus delaying optimal time of harvest and lowering the yields of infectious progeny. For example, it has been shown [24] that when a low MOI of an LGV biovar was added to HeLa cells, infected cells continued to replicate, and the chlamydial inclusion from these replicating cells remained in just one of the daughter cells, the other daughter escaping uninfected. In this way the number of uninfected cells may increase during the incubation period and a uniform population of mature EBs may never be realized. The replication of host cells, however, may be limited by addition of selective inhibitors (e. g., cycloheximide) to the infected cultures, thereby minimizing this problem.

When the proper conditions are established, intracellular RB replication generally proceeds for 2–3 days. During this time the chlamydiae synthesize their own DNA, RNA, and protein. They also elaborate glycogen-like polymers into the lumen of the vesicle, and this material begins to accumulate during the middle to late stages of inclusion development [25, 26]. The secretion of this extracellular polysaccharide is restricted to *C. trachomatis* strains and forms the basis of the iodine stain (glycogen stains dark brown), a widely used procedure to detect *C. trachomatis*-infected cells in culture. Continued RB replication eventually leads to the development of an intravacuolar microcolony that nearly fills the entire host cell cytoplasmic space. Development to this point is necessarily accompanied by an increase in the size of the inclusion membrane. Precisely how this occurs is not known, but new host protein synthesis is not required, since normal inclusion development occurs in the presence of cycloheximide, an inhibitor of eukaryotic protein synthesis. The origin of the initial endocytic vesicle is most certainly the host cell plasma membrane, but just how this membrane becomes modified as the infection proceeds is not clear. In this context, it has been observed that mitochondria establish a close relationship with the inclusion membrane. Matsumoto [27] showed, in transmission electron photomicrographs of isolated inclusion vesicles, that mitochondria often were seen physically bound to the cytoplasmic face of the inclusion membrane. Hatch [28] has shown that chlamydiae are dependent upon the host cell for intermediates of energy metabolism (ATP), and since ATP synthesis in eukaryotes occurs at the mitochondrion membrane, the close association of these respiratory organelles with chlamydial inclusions may very well be more than coincidental.

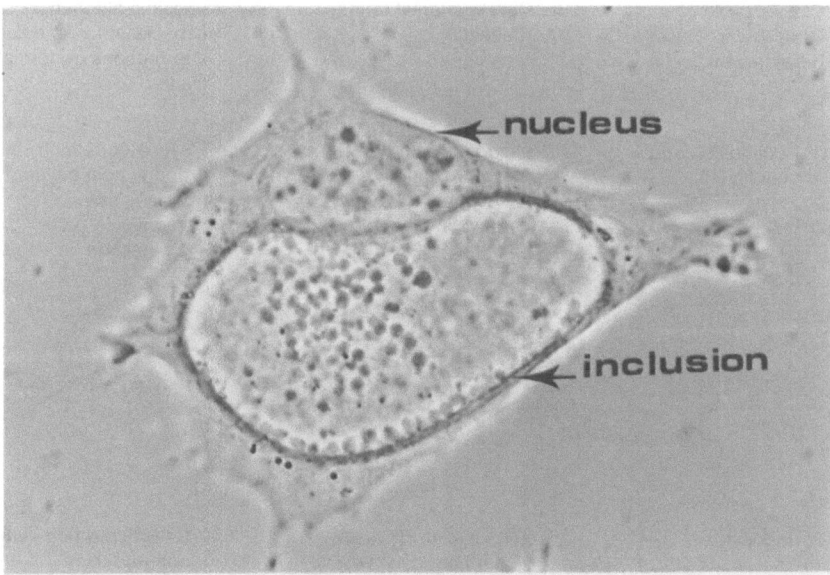

Fig. 6. A phase-contrast photomicrograph of a *C. trachomatis*-infected HeLa cell. The inclusion is filled not only with developing RBs, but also with glycogen. This structure stains purple with Giemsa and dark brown with iodine. (Photomicrograph by courtesy of Dr. C. D. Rothermel)

As the infectious cycle approaches completion, the large RB microcolony may actually contort the nucleus as it presses against it (Fig. 6). In time, RB replication diminishes, and once again EBs begin to appear as RB→EB differentiation becomes predominant. The molecular trigger for this round of differentiation is not known. The process is not perfectly synchronous. Some RBs differentiate fairly early (perhaps after a single day in culture), most rather late, and a few not at all. It is common to see developmental forms of intermediate morphology (transition forms) during the latter stages of the developmental cycle. At a point in the process when most RBs have converted to EBs, the inclusion membrane bursts and progeny EBs are released into the host cell cytoplasm. The host cell lyses soon after inclusion disaggregation, and a new generation of infectious EBs is released into the extracellular milieu, each one capable of initiating a new cycle of replication in a susceptible host cell. When conditions are ideal an increase of about 3 logs above the input multiplicity may be recovered at the end of the replicative cycle.

The details concerning intracellular chlamydial development have, to a large degree, been worked out in cell culture systems under carefully controlled conditions. When *C. trachomatis* infects epithelial cells in situ, giving rise to a polymorphonuclear inflammatory response or a mononuclear follicular inflammation [5], it is presumed that the cycle within the infected cell proceeds in an essentially similar manner. This in fact may be true in some instances, but a few basic differences between chlamydial development in cell cultures and naturally occurring infections should be noted. In cell cultures, the degree of infectivity can be precisely controlled, and conditions that establish successful passage have been standardized. In contrast,

Classic cycle of intracellular development	Developmental forms present	Possible alternatives, especially host-mediated interruptions of normal cycle
1. Recognition and attachment	elementary body (EB) gains proximity to susceptible host cell. The cycle may be initiated by a single EB	(a) EB may not attach properly host cell may be nonpermissive. Net: eradication prior to ingestion

nucleus

EB

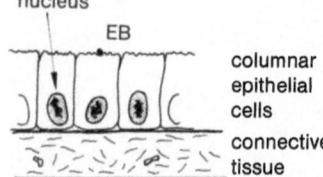

columnar epithelial cells

connective tissue

2. Endocytosis	intracellular EB within endocytic vesicle, fusion of lysosomes inhibited	(b) EB rendered non-viable during uptake Net: eradication prior to differentiation

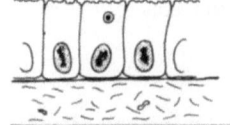

3. Differentiation	EB → reticulate body (RB) RB within membrane-bound vesicle	

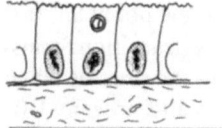

4. RB replication		(c) Reduced RB replication rates, possibly due to i) restriction of essential nutrients ii) Cytokine (interferon; lymphokine)-mediated host cell activation (mechanism not understood)

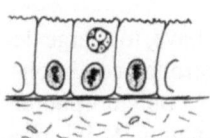

RB → RB → RB, RB → RB, RB → RB, RB → RB, RB → RB

RB growth by binary fissions, inclusion vesicle increases in size (mechanism unknown)

Net: prolonged RB (non-infectious) sequence, no cell to cell spread

Fig. 7. Schematic diagram of the developmental cycle of *C. trachomatis* in epithelial cells. Potential points of departure from the classic cycle and possible host-mediated interventions are indicated.

5. RB replication
   continues, EBs begin
   to appear

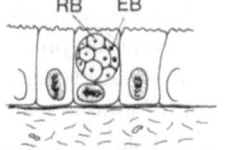

RB ↗ RB
RB ↗ ↘ RB
RB ↘ RB ↗ RB
RB ↘ RB

EB ⟶ RB

RB ↗ RB
RB ↗ ↘ RB
RB ↘ RB ↗ RB
RB ↘ RB

early RB → EB differentiation,
RB forms still predominate,
replication rates slow down

(d) interference with
    RB → EB
(e) slow-down of RB growth
    by above-mentioned
    mechanisms
(f) elaboration of extra-
    cellular antigen
    (e. g. polysaccharide) may
    lead to initation of
    inflammatory response,
    antibody production
    or both

6. RB -- RB differen-
   tiation

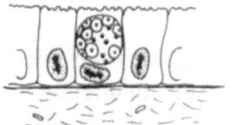

RB → EB
RB
RB → EB
RB → EB
EB
RB → EB
EBs predominate forms

7. Inclusion Membrance
   Lysis

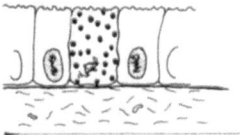

EBs free in Cytoplasm

(g) Infected host cell
    cytotoxicity apparent,
    possible iniation
    of inflammatory r x n
    (if not before)

(h) Immediate host cell
    cytotixicity due to
    large number of released
    EBs could occur.

8. Host cell lysis

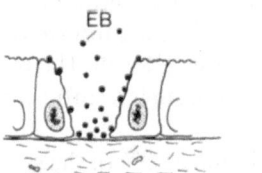

EBs released, initiating
of infectious cycle
may begin

(i) local or systemic
    spread may begin

(j) inflammatory rxn
    may begin here if
    not before

(k) antibody response may
    be triggered if not
    before

(l) host-mediated events
    could lead to irra-
    dication here or
    persistence in newly
    infected cells could
    occur

naturally occurring infections are most frequently characterized by the presence of only very few inclusions, and the associated tissue damage may be more related to the inflammatory response than to direct host cell destruction as a result of chlamydial growth and spread. The inflammatory phagocytes may serve to limit numbers of viable chlamydiae [29, 30] by acting as nonpermissive host cells. It is also possible that the cycle of chlamydial development in epithelial cells proceeds much less smoothly. For example, any interruption of the RB→EB differentiation phase would limit the numbers of infectious forms and decrease the possibility for spread to adjacent cells. There is some evidence that interferon [31] and other soluble lymphocyte mediators [32, 33] may act in precisely this way to limit chlamydial development. These concepts of microbiostatic mechanisms are corroborated by the histological aspects of chlamydial infections, and by the fact that normally very low yields of infectious chlamydiae are obtained from genital or ocular lesions, even in the presence of a demonstrable infection. Therefore, the laboratory models that stress either reduced chlamydial growth, interruption of RB→EB differentiation, or the presence of unique (noninfectious) forms of the organism [34] may more accurately reflect the true course of chlamydial development in infected individuals. A schematic diagram of the chlamydial developmental cycle, with potential alternative pathways, and possible combinations of host-mediated interventions, is outlined in Fig. 7.

An additional common complication of naturally occurring chlamydial infections is that mixed infections frequently occur. The study of mixed chlamydial infections has only recently been applied to laboratory investigation. Wyrick et al. [35] have shown that the presence of gonococci enhanced the intracellular development of a genital *C. trachomatis* strain in human cervical epithelial cell monolayers. Studies such as these will no doubt be expanded to include not only mixed bacterial infections *(Neisseria, Ureaplasma, Hemophilius)* but also mixed viral infections (herpesvirus, cytomegalovirus).

Metabolism

The enzymatic capabilities of replicating RBs have not been completely defined. Becker [8] has reviewed the biochemical potential of these parasites. They are capable of de novo nucleic acid and protein synthesis, possess a partial (non-energy-producing) sequence of glycolytic enzymes, synthesize and secrete glycogen [36], and metabolize lipids, producing some novel species [37]. Reticulate bodies utilize host cell nucleotide triphosphate pools, and these high-energy metabolites are transported into the chlamydial cell via an ATP-ADP exchange mechanism [38, 39]. The requirement for host-cell-generated intermediates of energy metabolism is a sufficient condition to render the chlamydiae obligatorily parasitic.

The chlamydial genome (about 6.6×10^8 daltons in size) is about 12% of the size of the *Escherichia coli* genome, and only three times the size of the T_4 bacteriophage genome [40]. The chlamydiae therefore have combined the translational products of their limited genetic information with available host cell metabolites to establish conditions which allow their replication at the expense of the host cell. A role for the inclusion membrane (whether mitochondrion or otherwise derived) in the processing of essential metabolites is also possible. It may be that the replicating RBs acting in concert with enzymatic activities present in this membrane serves as the functional unit of replication. All host-cell-derived or extracellular metabolites must be transported across this membrane before becoming available to RBs. A membrane-bound vesicle is most certainly not a requirement for intracellular parasitism per se, as the rickettsiae function quite well while growing free in the host cell cytoplasm or nucleus. If this membrane is required for chlamydial growth, then processing of nutrients and/or the selective transport of metabolites may be the function it provides. Definitive answers to these questions must await large-scale production of intact inclusions and purified inclusion membrane preparations. These studies have been attempted on several occasions but only recently have successful isolation procedures been accomplished [27].

The inclusion vesicle is also a highly osmotically stabilized environment. This fact partially explains why antibiotics that interrupt cell wall synthesis have not been successful in eradicating chlamydial infections. The effect of β-lactams on chlamydial development is a complex problem that also involves the unusual chemical composition of the chlamydial wall, but in the absence of a stabilized outer envelope, the osmotic environment provided by the inclusion vesicle represents a critical factor in the failure of penicillins and related antibiotics to control these microbes [42].

Antigens and Ultrastructure

A great deal of recent work has centered around defining the chlamydial antigens responsible for conferring genus, species, group, and type specificity, and for establishing relationships between the structural antigenic moieties and their function during chlamydial growth and development.

The genus-specific antigen has been recognized for decades, and forms the basis of the complement fixation test. The active antigenic determinant has been established as the 2-keto-3 deoxyoctanoic acid group of a complex acid polysaccharide [42].

Stuart and MacDonald [43] reported that a genus-specific polysaccharide antigen was elaborated into the culture medium of C. trachomatis-infected monkey kidney cells. This carbohydrate polymer was isolated in molecular weights ranging from 20000 to 200000 daltons, but for all molecular species tested, the material was composed of repeating units of a single monosaccharide. The specific moiety has not yet been identified, but aldetol acetate derivatives were eluted between the derivatives of glucose and galactose when analyzed by gas chromatography. It is well documented [26] that glycogen-like polysaccharides are elaborated into the inclusion of C. trachomatis-infected cells. The latter material has been identified by Garrett [25] as primarily composed of repeating glucose molecules joined principally by α-1,4-bonds, with α-1,6-linked branches. The average number of glucose units per acid-extractable chain was reported to be 16 ± 2, making the molecular weight range of the intrainclusional polysaccharide between 2500 and 3250 daltons. It therefore appears that the genus-specific carbohydrate polymer secreted into the medium is distinct from the glycogen within the vesicle. The presence of extracellular *C. trachomatis*-specific polysaccharides has not been documented in infected individuals, and their role in the inflammatory response to chlamydial infections is not known. If present, these antigens should be exploited as a diagnostic aid and investigated with respect to their inflammatory-mediating potential.

Caldwell et al. [44] found that *C. trachomatis* preparations from 24-h-infected HeLa cells, after nonionic detergent (Triton X-100) treatment, yielded 19 distinct precipitin lines in the soluble fraction when immunoelectrophoresed in a two-dimensional assay system using antisera raised in rabbits. Only one of the TX-100-soluble components cross-reacted with antisera raised against *C. psittaci*. However, when TX-100-soluble material was compared for trachoma and LGV strains of *C. trachomatis*, a striking similarity was observed in the precipitin patterns against heterologous sera. In a subsequent study, Caldwell et al. [45] demonstrated that a single TX-100-soluble antigen strongly cross-reacted with sera collected from individuals suffering from LGV, trachoma, chlamydial urethritis, and chlamydial cervicitis, but not psittacosis. This species-specific antigen (perhaps a membrane protein) is important in the serological diagnosis of chlamydial infections, since antibody against it can be detected in a variety of human *C. trachomatis* infections.

Serotype-specific antigens have also been isolated from *C. trachomatis* EB preparations. Sacks et al. [46, 47] reported that after mild (nonionic) detergent treatment, one of the proteins solubilized (molecular weight = 30 000 daltons) reacted exclusively with extensively adsorbed homologous antisera. Hourihan et al. [48], using molecular shift liquid chromatography, confirmed the specificity of the 30 000-dalton protein from a *C. trachomatis* serotype A isolate by measuring its shift to an appropriately elevated molecular weight after being bound by specific antibody. Study of the antigenic composition of chlamydiae has led to examination of functional relationships, especially at the surface of these organisms. When viewed by transmission electron microscopy, chlamydial EBs and RBs are enveloped within a trilaminar outer membrane similar in appearance to the outer envelope of gram-negative bacteria. Despite this apparent structural similarity, evidence of biochemical similarities have, until recently, not been observed. The chlamydial wall is distinct from other prokaryotes in that an electron-dense peptidoglycan layer is not present. This is in agreement with observations that have shown chlamydiae insensitive to lysozyme and lacking detectable quantities of *N*-acetylmuramic acid [49]. These studies suggest that chlamydiae do not contain the typical bacterial murein sheath that is believed to confer structural rigidity on the bacterial cell, yet chlamydial EBs still maintain a rigid external surface in its absence. Hatch et al. [50] and Caldwell et al. [51] have described a major outer membrane protein (MOMP) associated with the external envelope of *C. trachomatis* EBs. Thus the outer envelope of chlamydiae, like that of gram-negative bacteria, is composed primarily of a single major protein species. This protein (molecular weight 39 500 daltons) was isolated by Caldwell et al. [51] from a sarkosyl-treated insoluble EB preparation. Sarkosyl (a mildly anionic detergent) solubilized the majority of surface protein species from the outer envelope. The insoluble residue retained its structural integrity, and when subjected to sodium dodecyl sulfate (SDS) extraction yielded virtually quantitative amounts of MOMP. The MOMP reportedly comprised more than 60% of the outer envelope mass, and concomitantly with MOMP extraction, envelope structural integrity was lost. These data support the hypothesis that MOMP confers rigidity on the *C. trachomatis* cell. Matrix proteins (MOMP) from gram-negative bacteria are noncovalently linked to the peptidoglycan layer and contribute to the ultrastructure of transmembranous pores found in these organisms. Matsumoto and Higashi [52] recognized the presence of transmembranous structures in chlamydiae that originate on the inner face of the cytoplasmic membrane and interdigitate through to the external surface of the outer envelope. Several distinct protein species were proposed to compose the "pore-like" structure, and thus chlamydial MOMP may not only provide structural integrity to the outer envelope, but also serve as part of the pore-like assembly found in these organisms.

Despite the absence of chlamydial peptidoglycan, a tetrapeptide-linked matrix may very well be present. When penicillin or cycloserine is added to chlamydiae-infected cells, the usual cycle of development is interrupted. In addition, the presence of D-alanine competitively interferes with the action of cycloserine [53, 54], a further indication for the presence of tetrapeptide. In the presence of penicillin intracellular RBs are incapable of division, although macromolecular biosynthesis continues uninterrupted. The net result of continued biosynthesis in the absence of division is the formation of large, aberrant RB forms. Differentiation of RBs to EBs is also inhibited, and in this way the production of infectious progeny no longer occurs. The effects of penicillin on chlamydial growth have been most carefully studied with *C. psittaci* [55], but similar results have been reported for *C. trachomatis*-infected cells [56]. Barbour et al. [57] reported that three distinct penicillin-binding proteins (PBPs) were present in purified EB or RB preparations. The RBs quantitatively bound more penicillin, but the binding affinities of the drug were similar for EBs and RBs, implying that RB binding sites were more accessible than were EB binding sites. The binding of penicillin to EB PBPs reportedly had no effect on the initiation of infection, and the effect of bound penicillin was considerably reduced when the drug was deleted until late in the developmental cycle. When chlamydiae-infected cells were washed free of penicillin, normal development resumed subsequent to the reorganization of abnormal RB forms [55].

These studies collectively provide solid evidence that the structural rigidity of the *C. trachomatis* outer envelope makes it fundamentally distinct from eubacteria. The MOMP matrix of chlamydiae and gram-negative bacteria may be functionally and structurally analogous, but if D-alanine-containing tetrapeptides are present they are probably not cross-linked in a manner analogous to that observed in the gram-negatives (i.e., to a murein backbone).

Other Recent Developments

Our understanding of the molecular biology of chlamydiae is entering a new era. This is partially due to the influx of new researchers, but mostly due to the application of recent technological advances to the study of these microbes. For example, chlamydial genes are now being cloned in free living bacteria. Wenman and Lovett [58] have successfully established the presence of *C. trachomatis*-specific antigens in a lambda phage-transfected strain of *E. coli*.

Hybridoma cells that secrete monoclonal antibodies directed against a variety of *C. trachomatis* surface antigens were recently isolated [59], and these immunoglobulins are being tested as potential diagnostic reagents [60].

In other areas, Ward [61] has shown that regulation of chlamydial development may in part be governed by cyclic nucleotide levels. Ward also indicated the possibility that hormonal levels (especially the prostaglandins) may influence the course of infection in situ. Pearce and Allen [62] have reported a correlation between chlamydial amino acid requirements and the diseases most frequently associated with the various serotypes. For example, three serotypes that cause endemic trachoma (A, B, C) require the presence of exogenous tryptophan for growth in cell culture, whereas the genital strains (D-I) do not. The lipids of *C. trachomatis* EBs have been analyzed by Larsson et al. [63] using capillary gas chromatography. This sophisticated technique may not only lead to the discovery of fundamental distinctions between the two species and the various serotypes, but also could uncover unique properties associated with either the EB or the RB, and provide insight into the mechanisms of chlamydial differentiation. Finally, Hatch [38] is investigating the requirement for axenic chlamydial growth that would obviate the obligatory exigency of a eukaryotic host cell.

As work in these and other areas expands and continues we should soon be in a position more readily to diagnose, treat, and perhaps even prevent (at least some) chlamydial infections. This is not to say that we should become complacent. Recognition of additional infections of chlamydial etiology will no doubt be forthcoming, and therefore improved diagnostic and treatment protocols should continue to remain at the fore. But progress, like time and motion, is relative. Each depends on the point of view of the observer and for each it is important to note precisely where one stands. There are still fundamental questions concerning chlamydial-host cell interactions that remain unresolved. The subtle host-parasite checks and balances that constantly occur, and are critical to whether the infectious process results in overt parasite replication, persistence, or elimination, are not well understood. The chlamydia-animal cell systems that stress reduced parasite growth make excellent models for study of this problem. This question can also be generalized to a variety of other parasitic, bacterial, and viral infections using these same models. An additional poorly understood fundamental issue concerns the specific evolutionary adaptations that must have occurred to permit existence in an intracellular environment. This question is basic to the broader issue of how diverse species establish intimate associations, and may even relate to the subcellular organization. Progress concerning these basic issues may seem slow and fragmented, but after the chlamydial diseases have been recognized, categorized, and dealt with, these fundamental problems will remain and will keep students of chlamydiae busy for a long time to come.

Acknowledgments. Research in the author's laboratory is supported by Public Health Service Grant AI 19782 from the National Institute of Allergy and Infectious Diseases. I thank Alice Stapp, Caroline Fritsch, and Pat Hargraves for their assistance in the preparation of this manuscript.

References

1. Page LA (1974) Chlamydiales. In: Buchanan RE, Gibbons NE (eds) Bergey's manual of determinative bacteriology, 8th edn. Williams and Wilkins, Baltimore, pp 914-918
2. Moulder JW (1982) A primer for *Chlamydiae*. In: Mårdh P-A et al. (eds) Chlamydial infections. Elsevier Biomedical, Amsterdam, pp 3-14
3. Schachter J, Grossman M (1981) Chlamydial infections. Annu Rev Med 32: 45-61
4. Wang S-P, Grayston JT (1971) Classification of TRIC and related strains with micro immunofluorescence. In: Nichols RL (ed) Trachoma and related disorders caused by chlamydial agents. Excerpta Medica, Princeton, pp 305-321
5. Schachter J, Dawson C (1978) Human chlamydial infections. PSG, Littleton, pp 9-43
6. Darouger S, Treharne JD (1982) Cell culture methods for the isolation of *C. trachomatis* - a review. In: Mårdh P-A et al. (eds) Chlamydial infections. Elsevier Biomedical, Amsterdam, pp 265-274
7. Kingsbury DT, Weiss E (1968) Lack of deoxyribonucleic acid homology between species of the genus *Chlamydia*. J Bacteriol 96: 1421-1423
8. Becker Y (1978) The *Chlamydia:* molecular biology of procaryotic obligate parasites of eucaryocytes. Microbiol Rev 42: 274-306
9. Schachter J, Caldwell HD (1980) Chlamydiae. Annu Rev Microbiol 34: 285-309
10. Storz J, Spears C (1978) *Chlamydiales:* properties, cycle of development and effects on eucaryotic host cells. Curr Top Microbiol Immunol 76: 167-214
11. Kuo C-C, Wang S-P, Grayston JT (1973) Effect of polycations, polyanions, and neuraminidase on the infectivity of trachoma-inclusion conjunctivitis and lymphogranuloma venereum organisms in HeLa cells: sialic acid residues as possible receptors for trachoma-inclusion conjunctivitis. Infect Immun 8: 74-79
12. Soderlund G, Kihlstrom E (1982) Physicochemical surface properties of elementary bodies from different serotypes of *Chlamydia trachomatis* and their interaction with mouse fibroblasts. Infect Immun 36: 893-899
13. Byrne GI, Moulder JW (1978) Parasite-specified phagocytosis of *Chlamydia psittaci* and *Chlamydia trachomatis* by L and HeLa cells. Infect Immun 19: 598-606
14. Byrne GI (1978) Kinetics of phagocytosis of *Chlamydia psittaci* by mouse fibroblasts (L cells): separation of the attachment and ingestion stages. Infect Immun 19: 607-612
15. Sompolinsky D, Richmond S (1974) Growth of *Chlamydia trachomatis* in McCoy cells treated with cytochalasin B. Appl Microbiol 28: 912-914
16. Stirling P, Richmond S (1977) The developmental cycle of *Chlamydia trachomatis* in McCoy cells treated with cytochalasin B. J Gen Microbiol 100: 31-42
17. Lawn AM, Blythe WA, Taverne J (1973) Interaction of TRIC agents with macrophages and BHK-21 cells observed by electron microscopy. J Hyg (Lond) 71: 515-528
18. Gregory WW, Gardner M, Byrne GI, Moulder JW (1979) Arrays of hemispheric surface projections on *Chlamydia psittaci* and *Chlamydia trachomatis* observed by scanning electron microscopy. J Bacteriol 138: 241-244
19. Evans RT (1980) Suppression of *Chlamydia trachomatis* inclusion formation by fetal calf serum in cycloheximide-treated McCoy cells. J Clin Microbiol 11: 424-425
20. Evans RT, Taylor-Robinson D (1979) Comparison of various McCoy cell treatment procedures used for detection of *Chlamydia trachomatis*. J Clin Microbiol 10: 198-201
21. Evans RT, Taylor-Robinson D (1980) Detection of *Chlamydia trachomatis* in rapidly produced McCoy cell monolayers. J Clin Pathol 33: 591-594
22. LaScolea LJ Jr, Keddell JE (1981) Efficacy of various cell culture procedures for detection of *Chlamydia trachomatis* and applicability to diagnosis of pediatric infections. J Clin Microbiol 13: 705-708
23. Rota TR, Nichols RL (1973) *Chlamydia trachomatis* in cell culture. I. Comparison of efficiencies of infection in several defined media, at various pH and temperature values, and after exposure to diethylaminoethyl-dextran. Appl Microbiol 26: 560-565
24. Bose SK, Liebhaber H (1979) Deoxyribonucleic acid synthesis, cell cycle progression, and division of chlamydia-infected HeLa 229 cells. Infect Immun 24: 953-957

25. Garrett AJ (1975) Some properties of the polysaccharide from cell cultures infected with TRIC agent *(Chlamydia trachomatis).* J Gen Microbiol 90: 133-139

26. Gordon FB, Quan AL (1965) Occurrence of glycogen in inclusions of the psittacosis-lymphogranuloma venereum-trachoma agents. J Infect Dis 115: 186-196

27. Matsumoto A (1981) Isolation and electron microscopic observations of intracytoplasmic inclusions containing *Chlamydia psittaci.* J Bacteriol 145: 605-612

28. Hatch TP (1975) Utilization of L-cell nucleotide triphosphates by *Chlamydia psittaci* for ribonucleic acid synthesis. J Bacteriol 122: 393-400

29. Kuo C-C (1979) Interaction of *Chlamydia trachomatis* and mouse peritoneal macrophages. In: Schlessinger D (ed) Microbiology. ASM, Washington, pp 116-119

30. Yong EC, Klebanoff SJ, Kuo C-C (1982) Toxic effect of human polymorphonuclear leukocytes on *Chlamydia trachomatis.* Infect Immun 37: 422-426

31. Rothermel CD, Byrne GI, Havell EA (1982) Effect of fibroblast interferon on *Chlamydia trachomatis* replication in mouse fibroblasts (L cells). Infect Immun 39: 362-370

32. Byrne GI, Faubion CL (1982) Lymphokine-mediated microbistatic mechanisms restrict *Chlamydia psittaci* replication in macrophages. J Immunol 128: 469-474

33. Byrne GI, Faubion CL (1982) Lymphokine-mediated inhibition of *Chlamydia psittaci* replication in macrophages. In: Mårdh P-A, Holmes KK, Oriel JD, Piot P, Schachter J (eds) *Chlamydial infections.* Elsevier Biomedical, Amsterdam, pp 19-24

34. Moulder JW, Levy NJ, Shulman LP (1980) Persistent infection of mouse fibroblast (L cells) with *Chlamydia psittaci:* evidence for a cryptic chlamydial form. Infect Immun 30: 874-883

35. Wyrick PB, Sixby JW, Davis CH, Rump B, Walton LA (1982) Growth of *Chlamydia trachomatis* in human epithelial cell monolayers. In: Mårdh P-A et al. (eds) Chlamydial infections. Elsevier Biomedical, Amsterdam, pp 275-278

36. Weigent DA, Jenkin HM (1978) Contrast of glycogenesis and protein synthesis in monkey kidney cells and HeLa cells infected with *Chlamydia trachomatis* lymphogranuloma venereum. Infect Immun 20: 632-639

37. Fan VSC, Jenkin HM (1974) Lipid metabolism of monkey kidney cells (LLC-MK-2) infected with *Chlamydia trachomatis* strain lymphogranuloma venereum. Infect Immun 10: 464-470

38. Hatch TP (1982) Host free activities of *Chlamydia.* In: Mårdh P-A et al. (eds) Chlamydial infections. Elsevier Biomedical, Amsterdam, pp 25-28

39. Hatch TP, Al-Hossainy E, Silverman JA (1982) Adenine nucleotide and lysine transport in *Chlamydia psittaci.* J Bacteriol 150: 662-670

40. Kingsbury DT (1969) Estimate of the genome size of various microorganisms. J Bacteriol 98: 1400-1401

41. Kuo C-C, Wang S-P, Grayston JT (1977) Anti-microbial activity of several antibiotics and a sulfonamide against *C. trachomatis* in cell culture. Antimicrob Agents Chemother 12: 80-83

42. Dhir SP, Hakomori H, Kenny GE, Grayston JT (1972) Immunochemical studies on chlamydial group antigen (presence of a 2-keto-3-deoxycarbohydrate as immunodominant group). J Immunol 109: 116-122

43. Stuart ES, MacDonald AB (1982) Isolation of a possible group antigenic determinant of *Chlamydia trachomatis.* In: Mårdh P-A et al. (eds) Chlamydial infections. Elsevier Biomedical, Amsterdam, pp 57-60

44. Caldwell HD, Kuo C-C, Kenny GE (1975) Antigenic analysis of chlamydiae by two dimensional immunoelectrophoresis. J Immunol 115: 963-968

45. Caldwell HD, Kuo C-C, Kenny GE (1975) Antigenic analysis of chlamydiae by two-dimensional immunoelectrophoresis. II. A trachoma-LGV-specific antigen. J Immunol 115: 969-975

46. Sacks DL, MacDonald AB (1979) Isolation of a type-specific antigen from *Chlamydia trachomatis* by sodium dodecyl sulfate-polyacrylamide gel electrophoresis. J Immunol 122: 136-139

47. Sacks DL, Rota TR, MacDonald AB (1978) Separation and partial characterization of a type-specific antigen from *Chlamydia trachomatis.* J Immunol 121: 204-208

48. Hourihan JT, Rota TR, MacDonald AB (1980) Isolation and purification of a type-specific antigen from *Chlamydia trachomatis* propagated in cell culture utilizing molecular shift chromatography. J Immunol 124: 2399-2404

49. Garrett AJ, Harrison MJ, Manire GP (1974) A search for the bacterial mucopeptide component, muramic acid, in *Chlamydia.* J Gen Microbiol 80: 315-318

50. Hatch TP, Vance DW, Al-Houssainy E (1981) Identification of a major envelope protein in *Chlamydia* spp. J Bacteriol 146: 426–429
51. Caldwell HD, Kromhout J, Schachter J (1981) Purification and partial characterization of the major outer membrane protein of *Chlamydia trachomatis*. Infect Immun 31: 1161–1176
52. Matsumoto A, Higashi N (1975) Morphology of the envelopes of chlamydial organisms as revealed by freeze-etching techniques and scanning electron microscopy. Ann Rep Inst Virus Res Kyoto University 18: 51–61
53. Moulder JW, Novosel DL, Officer JE (1963) Inhibition of the growth of agents of the psittacosis group by D-cycloserine and its specific reversal by D-alanine. J Bacteriol 85: 707–711
54. Shiao LC, Wang S-P, Grayston JT (1967) Sensitivity and resistance of TRIC agents to penicillin, tetracycline, and sulfa drugs. Am J Ophthalmol 63: 1558–1568
55. Matsumoto A, Manire GP (1970) Electron microscopic observation on the effects of penicillin on the morphology of *Chlamydia psittaci*. J Bacteriol 101: 278–285
56. Johnson FWA, Hobson D (1977) The effect of penicillin on genital strains of *Chlamydia trachomatis* in cell culture. J Antimicrob Chemother 3: 49–56
57. Barbour AG, Amano KI, Hackstadt T, Perry L, Caldwell HD (1982) *Chlamydia trachomatis* has penicillin binding proteins but not detectable muramic acid. J Bacteriol 151: 420–428
58. Wenman WM, Lovett MA (1982) Cloning of *Chlamydia trachomatis* antigens recognized during human infections. In: Mårdh P-A et al. (eds) Chlamydial infections. Elsevier Biomedical, Amsterdam, pp 65–68
59. Stephens RS, Tom MR, Kuo C-C, Nowinski RC (1982) Monoclonal antibodies to *Chlamydia trachomatis:* antibody specificities and antigen characterization. J Immunol 128: 1083–1089
60. Tam MR, Stevens RS, Juo C-C, Holmes KK, Stamm WE, Nowinski RC (1982) Use of monoclonal antibodies to *Chlamydia trachomatis* as immunodiagnostic reagents. In: Mårdh P-A et al. (eds) Chlamydial infections. Elsevier Biomedical, Amsterdam, pp 317–320
61. Ward M (1982) Mechanisms governing HeLa cell susceptibility to chlamydial infection. In: Mårdh P-A et al. (eds) Chlamydial infections. Elsevier Biomedical, Amsterdam, pp 57–60
62. Pearce JH, Allen I (1982) Differential amino acid requirements of chlamydiae: regulation of growth and relationship with clinical syndrome. In: Mårdh P-A et al. (eds) Chlamydial infections. Elsevier Biomedical, Amsterdam, pp 29–32
63. Larsson L, Jimenez J, Odham G, Westerdahl G, Mårdh P-A (1982) Preliminary studies on cellular lipids of *Chlamydia trachomatis* using capillary gas chromatography. In: Mårdh P-A et al. (eds) Chlamydial infections. Elsevier Biomedical, Amsterdam, pp 37–40

Chlamydia Trachomatis:
Reiter's Syndrome and Reactive Arthritis

Andrew C. S. Keat

St. Stephen's Hospital, Fulham Road, Chelsea SW10 9TH, Great Britain

Introduction

In the last decade, substantial advances in microbiological techniques and human genetics have combined to provoke considerable interest in Reiter's syndrome (RS) and other forms of arthritis associated with infections. As a form of "reactive arthritis" the essential component of Reiter's syndrome is the apparent initiation of inflammatory joint and other musculoskeletal lesions by an infection at a site distant from the joint, though the inflammatory lesions themselves are sterile. Recognized precipitating infections include genital and gastro-intestinal infections, though it is likely that other types of "trigger" infection will also be identified. Other forms of reactive arthritis are associated with streptococcal tonsillitis or pharyngitis (rheumatic fever), and possibly tuberculosis (Poncet's disease), though these differ clinically and genetically from arthritis associated with genital or gut infection.

The importance of the reactive arthritides is three-fold. First, they represent one of the commonest forms of inflammatory joint disease amongst young adults throughout the world, and correct diagnosis is therefore essential for the management of a common and, at least transiently, disabling disorder. Second, and of perhaps greater significance, in reactive arthritis both genetic factors and the identity of some precipitating infectious agents are known, so that this condition may constitute a model for the study of tissue-damaging mechanisms in a wide variety of rheumatic and non-rheumatic disorders. Third, in a disease in which genetic predisposition can be identified and specific "triggering" infections are known, it may be possible to take steps for primary prevention or at least to prevent recurrences after an initial episode or arthritis.

The nomenclature and classification of this group of disorders is highly unsatisfactory. Certainly, the classic triad of Reiter's syndrome – arthritis, genital inflammation, and ocular inflammation – has a high discriminatory value. It is clear, however, that many patients have a similar disease but without all three criteria for the diagnosis of Reiter's syndrome. The existence of many patients with *formes frustes* has led to the description of the "Cheshire Cat syndrome" [1] to allude to those patients who by not conforming precisely to the strict confines of a clinical syndrome are excluded from precise categorization. This is problematic in both clinical practice and research studies.

Chlamydial Infections
Edited by P. Reeve
© Springer-Verlag Berlin Heidelberg 1987

Nomenclature and Classification of Reactive Arthritis

The term "Reiter's syndrome" was introduced in 1942 [2] to refer specifically to the triad of arthritis, genital inflammation, and ocular inflammation. The syndrome is sometimes expanded into a tetrad to include characteristic skin and mucous membrane lesions. When such ocular or mucocutaneous lesions are absent, the term "Reiter's disease" is frequently used. Many authors have expresses dissatisfaction with these terms and Hancock [3] noted at least 27 different terms which had at one time or another been introduced in their place. The two principal problems are that of finding a term which, by definition, includes patients with infection-triggered arthritis but who do not have the triad of Reiter's syndrome and that of devising a system of terminology which takes into account forms of seronegative arthritis which clinically resemble Reiter's syndrome and share the same genetic marker [4], but in which evidence of infection is lacking. Dissatisfaction with the terms "Reiter's syndrome" and "Reiter's disease" is amplified by the connotation of sexual promiscuity which they have unjustly acquired and by the fact that the contribution to this subject made by Hans Reiter [5] was small, far from novel, and in part erroneous.

Recently, two different approaches have been introduced to resolve the problems of nomenclature and classification of this group of seronegative arthritides. The introduction of the term "reactive arthritis" [6], whilst acknowledging the existence of a characteristic clinical entity, has shifted the basis of definition from the presence of certain clinical features to the relationship between a localized infection at one site and sterile synovitis (so far as can be demonstrated by conventional microbiological techniques) at another. Thus Dumonde and Steward [7] proposed that arthritis associated with infections should be classified as: (a) infective, when micro-organisms multiply within the joint, as in septic arthritis; (b) post-infective, when micro-organisms or microbial antigens are detected within the joint but do not multiply within the joint, as in meningococcal arthritis; (c) reactive, when there is infection at one site but no evidence of micro-organisms or of microbial antigens within the joint, as in rheumatic fever and Reiter's syndrome; and (d) inflammatory, when infection is suspected but no definite evidence as to the type or site of infection is available, as in rheumatoid disease. The distinction between post-infective and reactive arthritis may turn out to be spurious, as appropriate investigative techniques have yet to be thoroughly applied to conditions such as Reiter's syndrome.

An alternative clinical approach was introduced by Wright and Moll [8] in the concept of seronegative spondylarthritis. Recognition of clinical similarities between ankylosing spondylitis, Reiter's syndrome, enteropathic arthritis, psoriatic arthritis and Behçet's syndrome and observations that in family members of probands with one disease other diseases in the group occur with increased frequency led to this concept of a group of clinically and genetically interrelated conditions. To some extent, these interrelationships have been supported by the discovery of the high frequency of the HLA-B27 antigen in several members of the group.

From an aetiological viewpoint three subgroups of reactive arthritis can be recognized: sexually acquired arthritis, enterocolitic arthritis and reactive arthritis of unknown origin. In the last subgroup clinical and genetic features strongly suggest infection-triggered disease, though no evidence of infection can be detected (Fig. 1).

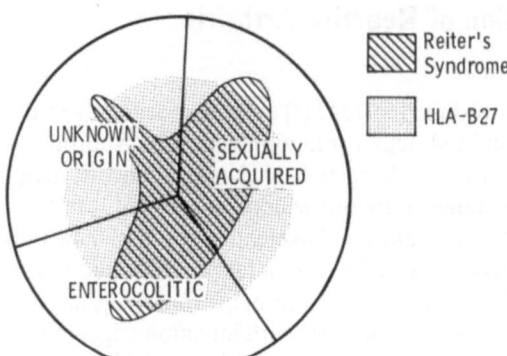

Fig. 1. Relationships between reactive arthritis, HLA-B27 and Reiter's syndrome.

In a proportion of patients in each group the triad of Reiter's syndrome is present. Since reactive arthritides are intimately related to other members of the seronegative spondylarthritis group, it is likely that in due course infectious triggers will also be found to operate in these conditions also. The position of rheumatic fever is somewhat anomalous, as although it is in some ways the archetype of reactive arthritis it does not fall within the seronegative spondylarthritis group. It differs both clinically and genetically from other forms of reactive arthritis and will not be discussed further.

Initiating Infections

In most parts of Europe and in the United States, genital infections are the commonest recognized initiators of reactive arthritis. Non-gonococcal genital infections (NGGI) are traditionally regarded as the only important group and there is abundant evidence that approximately 50% or more of cases of sexually acquired NGGI are caused by *Chlamydia trachomatis* infection. Gonococcal infection in reactive arthritis has been considered to be incidental, and indeed it is critical that a clear distinction be made between sterile reactive arthritis and the septic joint lesion of gonococcaemia. More recently, however, a possible role of gonococcal urogenital infections in the initiation of reactive arthritis has been considered [9]. It is of interest that other types of genital infection are also associated with the development of arthritis, though the relationship between arthritis and infection has been less intensively studied. A substantial proportion of patients with lymphogranuloma venereum (LGV) develop oligo-articular arthritis [10, 11], and sacro-iliitis has been reported in a high proportion of women with salpingitis [12, 13]. Findings of prostatitis in a high proportion of men with sacro-iliitis and spondylitis [14, 15] have been disputed and are of uncertain significance, as there are no hard criteria for the diagnosis of prostatitis. These conditions will not be considered further in this chapter.

Enteric infections by *Shigella flexneri* and *dysenteriae*, *Salmonella enteritidis* and *typhimurium*, *Yersinia enterocolitica* and *Campylobacter jejuni* have all been shown to lead to reactive arthritis in a minority of patients. *Shigella sonnei* infections are apparently devoid of this complication [16]. Early reports referred principally to the occurrence of arthritis during outbreaks of dysentery, though it is now clear that in many patients arthritis is preceded by a clinically trivial, short-lived illness. In a minority of patients symptoms of infection are absent even though culture or serological evidence of infection is obtained. Other gut infections, including giardiasis [17], amoebic dysentery [18] and non-specific traveller's diarrhea [19], have also been implicated in the induction of reactive arthritis, and joint lesions complicating short-circuit bowel operations in the treatment of obesity [20, 21] may also be regarded as reactive in nature. Because of the frequency of this complication, this kind of surgery is now seldom performed. Reactive arthritis associated with acute enteric infection should be distinguished from that associated with chronic inflammatory bowel disease [22, 23], and from that associated with Whipple's disease, in which micro-organisms may be present in the joints [24].

HLA-B27 Association

Following the dramatic demonstration that approximately 96% of patients with ankylosing spondylitis possess the histocompatibility antigen HLA-B27 [25, 26], the evident clinical interrelationships between spondylitis and Reiter's syndrome [27] led to the rapid demonstration of a similar, though less strong, association between the same antigen and Reiter's syndrome [28, 29]. No association with HLA-D locus antigens has been demonstrated. The calculated relative risk of developing Reiter's syndrome conferred by the possession of the B27 antigen ranges from 13-fold to 178-fold, depending to a considerable extent upon the selection criteria used in in-

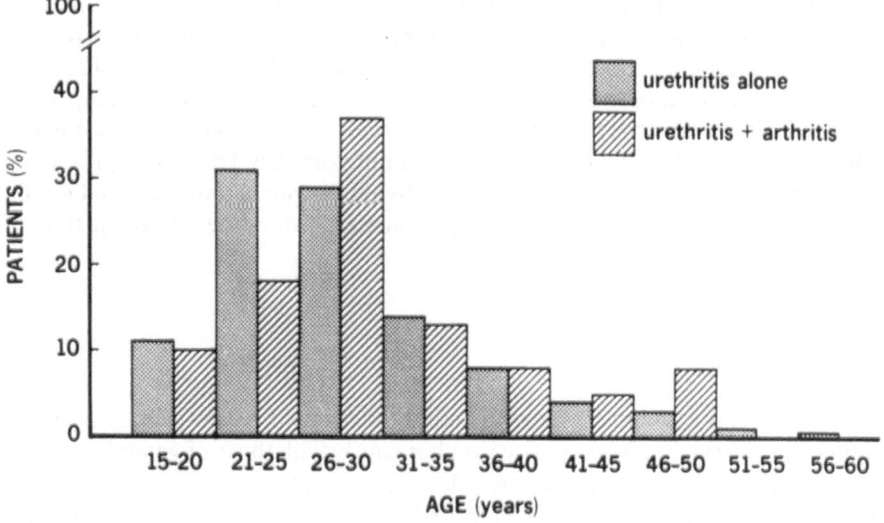

Fig. 2. Age incidence of sexually acquired reactive arthritis and non-gonococcal urethritis.

dividual studies [30, 31]. It is now clear that B27 positivity predisposes to the development of arthritis in certain forms of genital and enteric infections, though it does not affect the outcome of streptococcal [32], meningococcal [33] or certain viral infections [34]. It is also important that three other groups of patients – those with seronegative peripheral oligo-arthritis without evidence of infection, those with isolated calcaneodynia and tendonitis [35] and those with acute anterior uveitis, irrespective of the presence of associated rheumatic disease [36, 37] – also share a high prevalence of the HLA-B27 antigen. Thus the same genetic factor appears to be associated with a number of different entities, which can occur together in the same individual or in different members of a family [38, 39]. It is postulated that these other conditions not associated with overt infection may nevertheless also be initiated by infectious agents.

The significance of the HLA-B27 antigen in the pathogenesis of reactive arthritides is a source of considerable controversy. The role of genetic factors in the pathogenesis of reactive arthritis is fully discussed elsewhere [39–41].

Clinical Features

Epidemiology

Reactive arthritis of most commonly affects individuals in the third decade of life. The age incidence of arthritis associated with sexually acquired genital infection closely mirrors that of uncomplicated non-gonococcal urethritis (NGU) (Fig. 2), though that following enteric infections occurs not infrequently in children and older adults. The true sex ratio is difficult to calculate precisely, as Reiter's syndrome has traditionally been regarded as a male disease and many cases associated with dysentery have occurred in epidemics affecting predominantly male military personnel. However, available evidence indicates that arthritis occurs equally in males and females after enteric infections, though males predominate by approximately ten to one when genital infection is the trigger. Estimates of the incidence of reactive arthritides are also imprecise, as it is clear that many individuals develop mild, short-lived disease and may not present themselves for medical attention. Figures gathered from hospital attenders suggest that approximately 1% of men presenting with sexually acquired NGU and 2.5% of individuals with certain bacterial gut infections develop reactive arthritis [42]. Approximately 30% of these have the triad of Reiter's syndrome.

Presentation

Medical attention is frequently sought initially because of genito-urinary or bowel symptoms. Joint symptoms may arise simultaneously with those of genital or gut infection, and occasionally arthritis precedes evidence of infection; in 90% of patients, however, synovitis develops within 30 days of the onset of symptoms of infection, with a mean of 14 days. The incubation period of sexually acquired NGU is approximately 8–15 days, so that in individuals with sexually acquired reactive arthritis (SARA) the mean overall putative incubation period is approximately 28 days. In some individuals with SARA the interval between infection and arthritis may be much longer; in these patients there may be a period of latent or subclinical infection which is allowed to recrudesce by changes in the patients' immune status. Acute peripheral arthritis, commonly in the knee or small joints of the feet, is usually the first rheumatic symptom, though presentation may be precipitated by painful tenosynovitis, enthesopathy or low back pain. It is not uncommon for considerable knee effusions to be ignored by patients, or attributed to trivial injuries, but the presence of bilateral knee synovitis or of other characteristic lesions, especially at entheses, the junctional areas between tendon or fascia and bone, points to the correct diagnosis. Occasionally, a family history of spondylitis, episodic peripheral arthritis or acute anterior uveitis, will also give a helpful diagnostic clue.

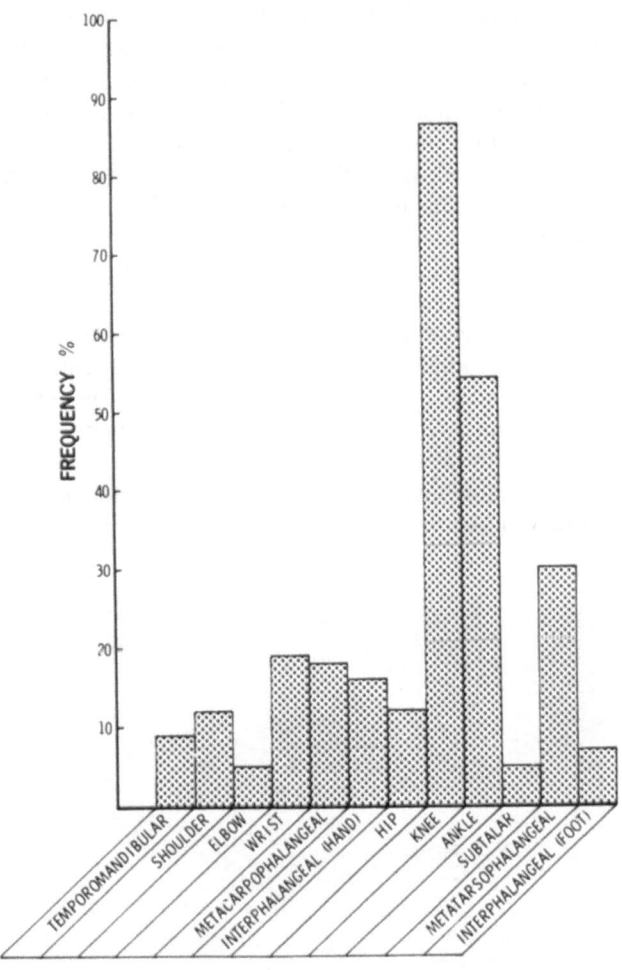

Fig. 3. Pattern of joint involvement in reactive arthritis.

Arthritis

In 50% of patients the knee joint is the first site to be affected, the ankle, metatarso-phalangeal joints and wrist being also commonly involved early in the course of disease. The full picture of joint disease generally evolves over 2–3 weeks, it being unusual for new sites to become affected after this time. Approximately 10% of patients remain with mono-arthritis, usually of a knee, ankle or wrist: the remainder develop oligo-articular disease, When small joints are affected, characteristically only one or two of the group (e. g. metatarsophalangeal joints) are involved, in contrast to the typical involvement of all joints in the group in rheumatoid disease. The pattern of joints affected in SARA is shown in Fig. 3. Persistence of synovitis may lead to articular erosions, especially where small joints are concerned (Fig. 4). The large joints usually remain radiographically normal, although juxta-articular osteoporosis may be noted. Synovial fluid examination in the acute phase usually reveals a turbid inflammatory exudate rich in polymorphonuclear leucocytes. This procedure is important for the exclusion of bacterial joint infection and crystal synovitis, though does not yield other specific diagnostic information. Synovial biopsy also reveals little diagnostically useful information, there being non-specific patchy inflammatory cell infiltrates in the subsynovium. Appearances may be indistinguishable from those in rheumatoid disease. Immunofluorescence studies of synovial biopsies obtained within the first few weeks of disease have shown the presence of immunoglobulin and complement C3 deposits consistent with the deposition or local formation of immune complexes [43, 44].

Low back pain is common during the acute episode. The exact cause of this cannot usually be established, though in many instances the signs and symptoms are strongly suggestive of sacro-iliitis. The proportion of patients developing radiographic sacro-iliitis varies considerably from one study to another: this is accounted for, in the main, by patient selection and duration of follow-up, definite radiographic sacro-iliitis being present in 5%–10% of patients with active acute disease [45–47], but in up to 50% of those having had continuous symptoms for 5 years or more [48–50]. Radionuclide scintigraphy using technetium-99m-polyphosphate has been employed as a means of detecting mild or early sacro-iliitis before radiographic

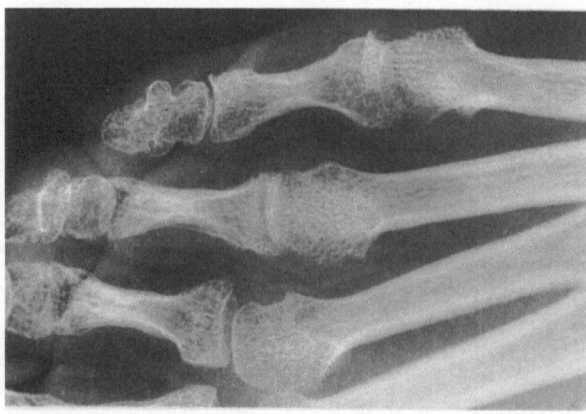

Fig. 4. Articular erosions at metatarsophalangeal joints.

changes have developed [51, 52]; on the basis of this technique, it has been suggested that acute sacro-iliitis occurs in approximately two-thirds of patients with Reiter's syndrome [53].

Reactive Arthritis and Spondylitis

The question as to whether reactive arthritis leads on to spondylitis remains controversial. Good [54] drew attention to development of ankylosing spondylitis in 12 of 35 (34%) men with Reiter's syndrome followed up for 2 years; other studies [55, 56] have suggested a much lower incidence, though Sairanen and colleagues [57] noted the presence of spondylitis in 32 of 100 of Paronen's 344 cases [58] when these were reviewed many years after the original episode. However, spondylitis and reactive arthritis may occur in different members of the same family, and several studies have suggested that up to 20% of HLA-B27-positive individuals will develop spondylitis [59, 60]. Thus in a group of 100 patients with reactive arthritis, of whom 75% were HLA-B27 positive, 14 might be expected to develop spondylitis also. However, the position is undoubtedly more complex than this. Recent family studies [60a, 60b] have indicated that HLA-B27-positive relatives of patients with ankylosing spondylitis are approximately twice as likely to develop the disease as unrelated, randomly selected HLA-B27-positive individuals. This suggests that HLA-B27-positive spondylitics possess (an)other genetic factor(s) besides HLA-B27, which also contribute(s) to the development of disease. It remains to be seen whether non-HLA-B27 genes associated with reactive arthritis also predispose to the development of ankylosing spondylitis. It has been speculated [61, 62] that features of reactive arthritis and spondylitis may be determined by separate, though closely linked, genetic factors in or close to the major histocompatibility complex which may be inherited separately or in various combinations and which may be activated by different "trigger" mechanisms.

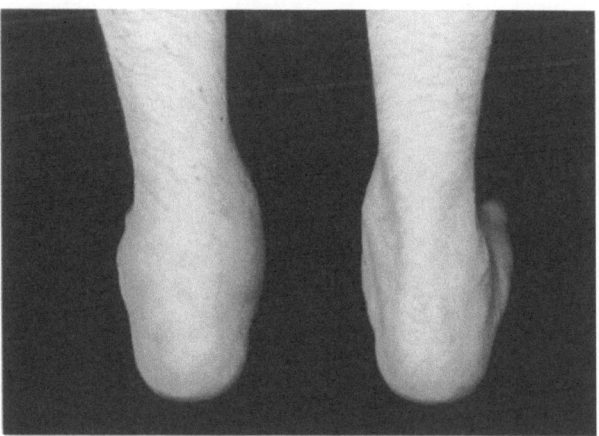

Fig.5. Achilles tendon bursitis.

Other Musculoskeletal Lesions

Inflammatory lesions at entheses [63, 64] are highly characteristic of reactive arthritis and often clinically troublesome. These occur in approximately 30% of patients and may also be present in other forms of seronegative arthritis. The sites of attachment of the plantar fascia and Achilles tendon to the calcaneum are most commonly involved: these lesions are characterized clinically by localized tender swellings and they may appear on the radiograph as bony erosions. There may be associated Achilles tendon bursitis (Fig. 5). Muscle and tendon attachments at the base of skull, pelvis, tibial tubercle, and feet may also be affected. Enthesopathic lesions heal with the formation of fluffy periosteal outgrowths with characteristic appearances at the pelvis (Fig. 6) and plantar calcaneal spurs. Tenosynovitis also occurs in a minority of patients, most commonly at the wrist extensors and foot dorsiflexors, and digital tendon expansion synovitis (sausage digit; Fig. 7) is uncommon but highly characteristic of this group of conditions. This may be associated with periostitis of the underlying bone.

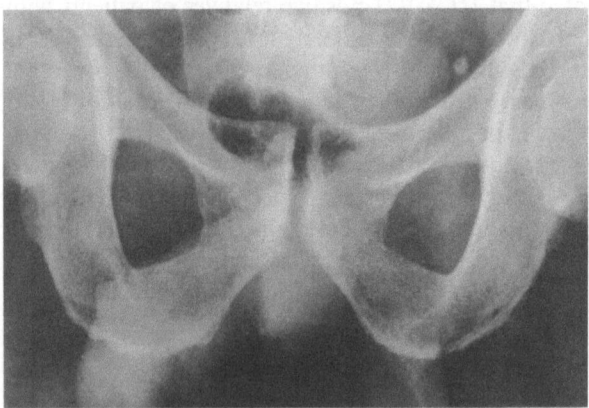

Fig. 6. Fluffy periosteal reaction in the pelvis of a young man.

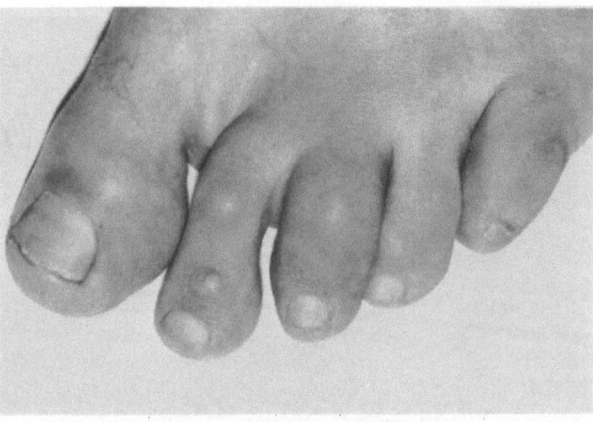

Fig. 7. Digital tendon expansion synovitis (sausage digit).

Mucous Membrane and Skin Lesions

Several mucous membrane and skin lesions are characteristic of reactive arthritis. Approximately 10% of patients develop keratoderma blennorrhagica, a scaling pustular rash on the soles of the feet (Fig. 8), and a similar proportion of patients develop circinate balanitis (Fig. 9). Circinate psoriasiform lesions have also been described on the female genitalia (Fig. 10) [65]. The lesions are histologically indistinguishable from those of pustular psoriasis [66, 67]. Painless oral ulcers are also not uncommon, in contrast to the extremely painful lesions of Behçet's syndrome, and the tongue may also be involved. Rarely, psoriatic skin lesions may be present elsewhere, and in the absence of other characteristic lesions of Reiter's syndrome it may be impossible to distinguish reactive arthritis from psoriatic arthritis with certainty. Psoriasis is closely associated with the HLA antigens B13, B17 and CW6. No such association has, however, been shown in patients who have these skin and mucous membrane lesions together with reactive arthritis [68]; instead, these lesions tend to occur in B27-positive-individuals, and in one study of nine men with isolated circinate balanitis, eight were shown to be HLA-B27 positive [69]. Circinate balanitis is common in reactive arthritis associated with *Shigella* dysentery [58], though no psoriasiform lesions have been recorded in reactive arthritis associated with other enteric infections. In *Yersinia* arthritis erythema nodosum occurs in a small proportion of cases and urticarial skin rashes have also been described [70].

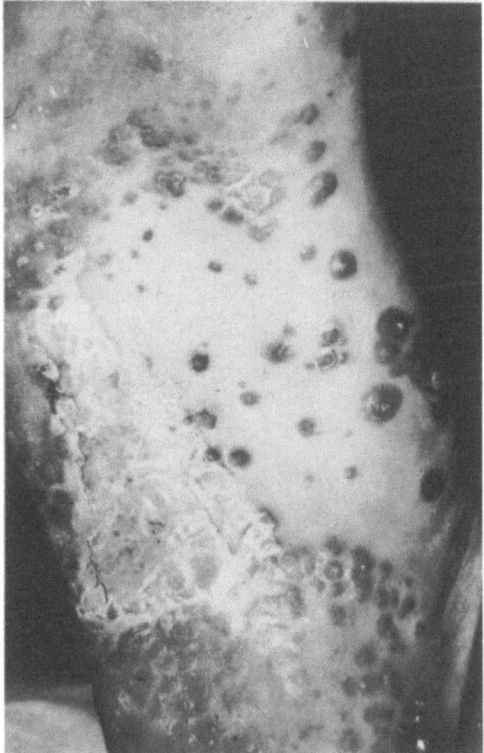

Fig. 8. Keratoderma blennorrhagica on the sole. (Courtesy of Dr. Brian Evans)

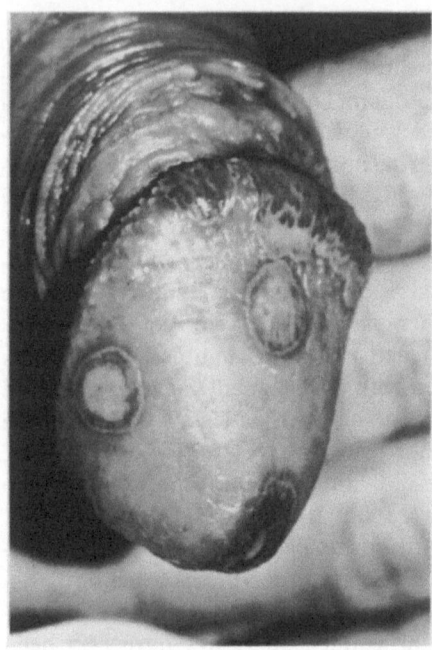

Fig. 9. Circinate balanitis. (Courtesy of Dr. Brian Evans)

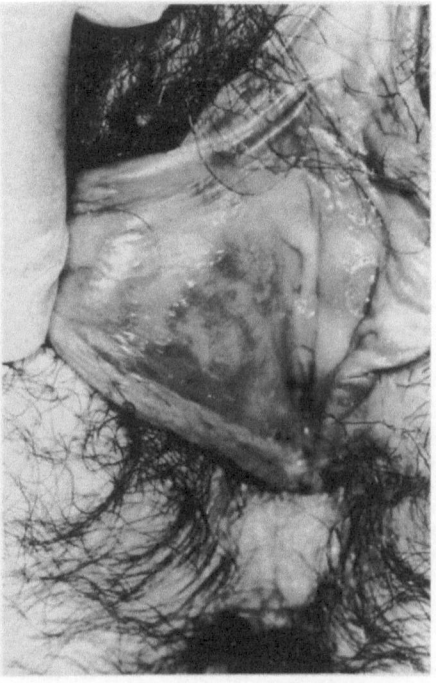

Fig. 10. Circinate vulvitis. (Courtesy of Dr. Isaac Thambar)

Ocular Lesions

Ocular inflammation is regarded as an essential constituent of the triad of Reiter's syndrome, though only a third to a half [46, 68] of patients with reactive arthritis are shown to have this feature. The frequency of conjunctivitis in different reported series partly reflects the vigour with which it is sought and its use as a diagnostic criterion. It is usually a mild, transient problem requiring no specific therapy. Acute anterior uveitis (AAU) occurs rarely during the acute episode of arthritis, though a history of this is given by approximately 4% of patients [42]. The occurrence of AAU in the past or family history of patients presenting with arthritis may give a valuable diagnostic clue. The distinction between conjunctivitis and AAU is often impossible to make without a specialist examination, and in view of the potentially rapid onset of blindness in this condition all patients with painful red eyes should be examined urgently by an ophthalmologist. Other ocular lesions, including keratitis [68, 71], retinitis [72], intraocular haemorrhage [58, 73] and hypopyon [74], have also been noted.

Other Systemic Lesions

Electrocardiographic evidence of carditis is present in 5%–13% of individuals with reactive arthritis, irrespective of the type of initiating infection [42]. This is usually restricted to some conduction delay manifesting as prolongation of the P-R interval, though occasionally arrhythmias may occur. This may give rise to considerable diagnostic difficulty, as the disease may closely resemble rheumatic fever [75]. Transient systolic murmurs have also been described [76, 77] and pericarditis may rarely be detected [78]. Carditis is rarely clinically evident and seldom gives rise to long-term cardiac disease. Approximately 1% of patients, generally those with long-standing, aggressive disease, develop aortic valve disease and some patients have undergone successful valve replacement [79]. No other cardiac valve defects have been described.

Neurological lesions occur rarely and the nature of their association with reactive arthritis remains uncertain. Widespread brain-stem lesions with multiple cranial nerve involvement [80] and Guillain-Barré syndrome [70] have been described, and optic neuritis [71, 81] and retrobulbar neuritis [82] also rarely occur. Myositis was reported in two of 74 patients with *Yersinia* arthritis [70], and pleurisy [58] and amyloidosis [83] have also been noted as rare complications.

Clinical Course

In the majority of patients, localization of all rheumatic and extra-articular lesions occurs within 3 weeks of the onset. Joint involvement is relatively constant, in contrast to the migratory arthritis or arthralgia of rheumatic fever and gonococcal arthritis. Symptoms generally subside over 3–5 months, 70% of patients showing complete resolution of disease within 6 months. In 5%–15% of patients, symptoms persist for longer than 1 year, and some of these patients run a relapsing and remitting course for several years. Approximately one in five patients with arthritis associated with genital infection will suffer one or more recurrences of rheumatic symptoms, though this may be restricted to tendonitis, bursitis or enthesopathy. Recurrence is not always associated with evidence of genital inflammation or further sexual contact, and conversely individuals who have suffered from reactive arthritis in the past may develop undoubted venereal urethritis without recurrence of their joint disease.

Treatment

There is no firm evidence that treating the precipitating infection influences the course of arthritis. However, it is clearly sensible practice to treat genital infection in both the patient and sexual partner(s) with appropriate antibiotics. Enteric infections are usually best managed without antibiotics unless septic complications arise. Rheumatic symptoms generally respond well to non-steroidal anti-inflammatory drugs, though heel enthesopathies may be very resistant and disabling. Judicious local injections of corticosteroids may be valuable in plantar fasciitis, though are not recommended for Achilles tendon lesions because of the danger of rupture of the tendon. Similarly, acute knee synovitis may be greatly helped by a local steroid injection, provided that appropriate steps have been taken to exclude joint infection. Systemic steroid therapy may be useful in patients with very severe extensive disease, though is less predictably effective than in rheumatoid disease and is usually unnecessary. Cytotoxic drugs including methotrexate may be effective in severe cases, but the "antirheumatoid" drugs penicillamine and gold have little or no effect. Bed rest or local splinting is desirable when joints are acutely inflamed, though most patients may be kept ambulant throughout the acute episode.

Physical measures may be of considerable help, especially the provision of heel pads when there is plantar fasciitis or Achilles tendonitis and insoles with metatarsal cushions when there is troublesome synovitis at the metatarsophalangeal joints. Ocular lesions require urgent assessment by an ophthalmologist and anterior uveitis should be treated with topical steroid drops. Skin lesions usually respond to topical applications of salicylic acid or hydrocortisone. Cardiac conduction defects do not generally require any specific therapy, though rarely surgical replacement of the aortic valve has been performed.

Prognosis

Most patients with reactive arthritis recover completely with no sequelae and no significant residual disability. Several authors have alluded to the serious outlook for patients with classic Reiter's syndrome [57, 84, 85]. It is important, however, that these studies have tended to select patients with severe joint and extra-articular lesions, and may have excluded many patients with only transient symptoms and limited disease. Such patients may not seek the advice of a rheumatologist, or may not have fulfilled existing criteria for inclusion in the studies. It is becoming clear that, in patients with reactive arthritis, HLA-B27 positivity is associated with more severe joint disease, the presence of extra-articular lesions and a longer disease course [86–88]. Thus patients with classic Reiter's syndrome with ocular and other associated lesions are likely to be HLA-B27 positive and to have a less favourable outcome than those with less extensive disease, a high proportion of whom will be B27 negative, and who may anticipate complete recovery.

Chlamydial Infection

Evidence from human genital infections and certain forms of animal arthritis suggest that chlamydial genital infection may be important in the initiation of reactive arthritis. Since the very early work of Lindner [89], overwhelming evidence has accrued that *Chlamydia trachomatis* infection is the cause of a high proportion, probably in excess of 50% of cases of non-gonococcal urethritis. In view of the known genetic susceptibility of individuals who develop reactive arthritis, it is possible that this infection could trigger off arthritis in the small group of susceptible individuals. It is also well recognized that disseminated chlamydial infection in sheep and calves [90, 91] may produce a severe polyarthritis sometimes associated with conjunctivitis and other systemic lesions. This condition clearly resembles, albeit superficially, Reiter's syndrome [92]. It has been demonstrated that arthritis can be induced in animal models by the injection of chlamydiae into the joints [93], though the relevance of these studies to human arthritis remains uncertain.

In those with SARA, culture and immunological data indicate that approximately 50% of patients have acute *C. trachomatis* genital infection at the onset of symptoms. Few data are available on reactive arthritis associated with extra-genital infections.

Genital Tract Infection and Reiter's Syndrome

Siboulet and Galestin [94] first isolated a chlamydia-like agent from the genital tract of men with Reiter's syndrome, and these findings were supported by other workers using ovoculture or light microscopy of Giemsa-stained preparations of urethral exudate (Table 1). More consistent data have been obtained since the introduction of the McCoy cell culture system; in Finnish [95] and British series [96], urethral isolates of *C. trachomatis* were obtained from 69.2% and 36% respectively of patients with acute reactive arthritis with active genital inflammation (Table 1).

Joint Infection and Reiter's Syndrome

The question as to whether viable chlamydiae enter the joint is of critical importance but remains unresolved. Isolates from synovial fluid and synovium were reported by several groups of workers using ovoculture techniques (Table 2); these findings have not been confirmed by other workers using the McCoy cell culture

Table 1. Isolation of *Chlamydia trachomatis* from the genital tract in patients with sexually acquired Reiter's syndrome or reactive arthritis

Author	Date	No. of patients	No. positive (%)	Culture technique
Siboulet and Galestin [94]	1962	3	3	Ovoculture
Schachter [108]	1976	81	12 (14.8)	Ovoculture
Delbarre and Amor [109]	1976	101	73 (72.3)	Light microscopy (Giemsa)
Dunlop et al. [110]	1968	20	2 (10)	Ovoculture
Ford [111]	1968	12	0	Ovoculture
Ford and McCandlish [112]	1971	14	0	McCoy cell culture
Vaughan-Jackson et al. [113]	1972	10	3 (33.3)	McCoy cell culture
Gordon et al. [114]	1973	1	1	McCoy cell culture
Kousa et al. [95]	1978	52	36 (69.2)	McCoy cell culture
Keat et al. [96]	1980	25	9 (36.0)	McCoy cell culture
Vilppula et al. [103]	1981	31	5 (16.1)	McCoy cell culture

Table 2. Isolation of *Chlamydia trachomatis* from synovial fluid (SF) and synovium (Sy) in patients with sexually acquired Reiter's syndrome or reactive arthritis

Author	Date	No. of patients	No. positive	SF/Sy	Culture technique
Schachter [108]	1976	81	6	SF 4/34 Sy 5/29	Ovoculture
Delbarre and Amor [109]	1976	50	33	Sy	Ovoculture
Dunlop et al. [110]	1968	4	4	SF 3 Sy 1	Ovoculture
Shatkin et al. [115]	1973	1	1	SF	Ovoculture
Gordon et al. [114]	1973	12	0	SF 0/12	McCoy cells
Harisijades et al. [116]	1975	20	0	SF	Ovoculture
Harisijades et al. [116]	1975	10	0	SF	McCoy cells
Keat and Thomas, unpublished results	1980	20	0	SF	McCoy cells

technique and the findings of one group have been retracted. However, maintaining cell cultures in the presence of synovial fluid presents particular problems, so that further work remains to be done before this crucial issue can be resolved.

Ocular Infection and Reiter's Syndrome

The genital tract is well known as a reservoir of infection in individuals with inclusion conjunctivitis [97]. Dawson and colleagues [98] obtained immunofluorescent evidence of local chlamydial ocular infection in 18% of a group of patients with Reiter's syndrome who also had other evidence of chlamydial infection elsewhere. Again, culture studies using the McCoy cell system have so far failed to confirm these findings (Table 3).

Table 3. Isolation of *Chlamydia trachomatis* from the eyes of patients with sexually acquired Reiter's syndrome or reactive arthritis

Author	Date	No. of patients	No. positive (%)	Culture technique
Dawson et al. [98]	1970	24[a]	5 (18)	Immunofluorescence
Schachter [108]	1976	33	3 (9.1)	Ovoculture
Gordon et al. [114]	1973	12	0	McCoy cells
Keat and Ridgway, unpublished results	1980	6	0	McCoy cells

[a] All patients considered to have chlamydial infection by criteria of positive culture at at least one site or complement fixation test antibody titre 1: ⩾ 16

Serological Studies and Reiter's Syndrome

As with culture data, improved serological techniques for the detection of specific chlamydial antibody render results obtained more than a decade or so ago especially difficult to interpret. Since the introduction of the micro-immunofluorescence (MIF) technique [99] some inconsistencies still occur, some workers using single or pooled antigens whilst others use multiple antigen techniques. In either case, however, the increased sensitivity of the MIF technique is maintained over the older complement fixation techniques (CFT). Using a CFT, Schachter and colleagues [100] found raised titres of chlamydial antibody in the serum of five of 16 (33%) pat-

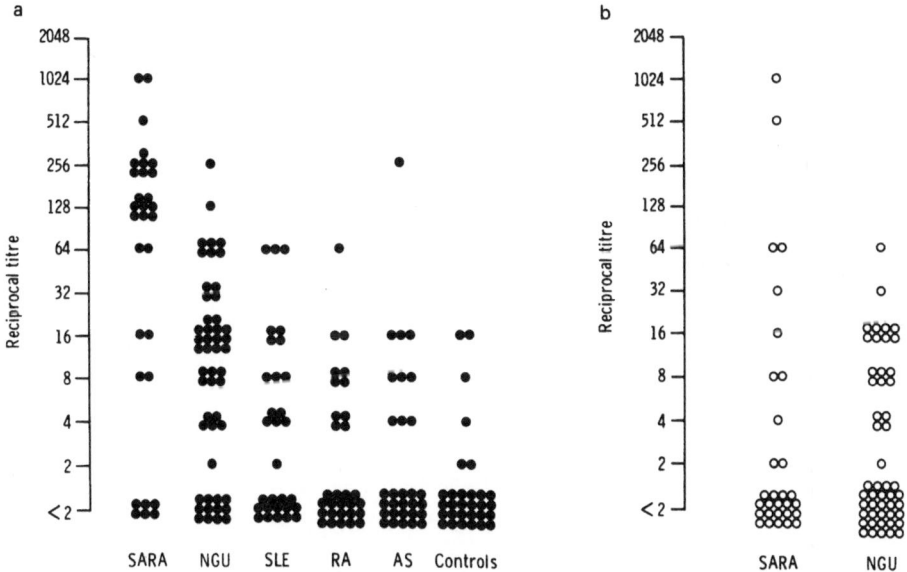

Fig. 11 a, b. Titres of **a** IgG and **b** IgM chlamydial antibody in serum of patients with sexually acquired reactive arthritis *(SARA)*, non-gonococcal urethritis (NGU), systemic lupus erythematosus *(SLE)*, rheumatoid arthritis *(RA)* and ankylosing spondylitis *(AS)* and in that of healthy controls [96].

ients with Reiter's syndrome. Kinsella, Norton and Ziff [101] found essentially similar results using a CFT (with an antigen derived from a *Chlamydia* strain capable of producing arthritis in sheep) with raised titres of serum antibody in nine of 24 (37.5%) patients with Reiter's syndrome: they obtained almost identical results in men with uncomplicated NGU, though raised titres were found only in 8% of normal controls and in none of a group of patients with ankylosing spondylitis. Dawson and colleagues [98], also using CFT, studied 24 patients with Reiter's syndrome who had culture or serological evidence of chlamydial infection and a group of patients with inclusion conjunctivitis (IC): half of the patients with IC and 75% of those with Reiter's syndrome had raised titres of chlamydial antibody, and the authors noted that whilst titres never rose above 1:32 in IC patients, eight of 24 individuals with Reiter's syndrome had titres between 1:64 and 1:256.

With the introduction of the MIF method, Darougar [102] noted raised titres of immunofluorescent antibody in 77% of 18 patients with Reiter's syndrome, though with a geometric mean titre (GMT) of 26, substantially lower than that found in patients with lymphogranuloma venereum or psittacosis. These titres were similar in frequency and level to results obtained from men with uncomplicated NGU. However, the duration or degree of activity of arthritis in these patients was not described and it may be significant that an isolate was not obtained from the genital tract in any of them. Kousa and colleagues [95], using a single-antigen MIF test, demonstrated serum titres of chlamydial antibody 1: ⩾8 in 79 of 91 men with Reiter's syndrome (87%), compared with six of 25 (24%) of the controls. In this study an anti-whole human immunoglobulin was used, so that data relating to the immuno-

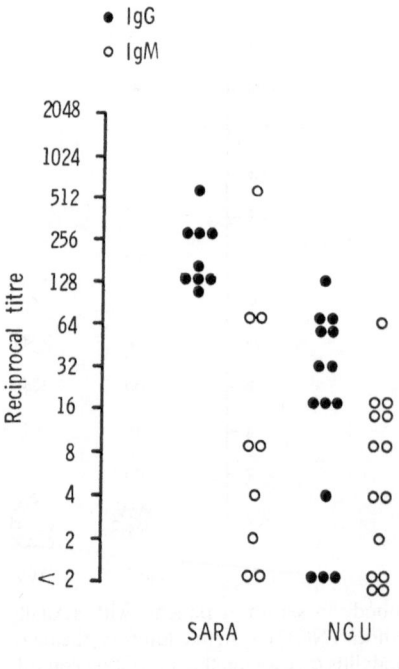

Fig. 12. Titres of IgG and IgM chlamydial antibody in isolate-positive and -negative patients with SARA and NGU [96].

globulin class were not obtained. The GMT of serum antibody in these patients was 69, and it was noted that titres were higher in patients with a disease duration of less than 3 months and in those with positive urethral cultures. Essentially similar results were obtained by Keat and colleagues [96], though in this prospective study of 30 male patients all of whom had early disease, a slightly lower GMT of 47.5 was found. In this study, using a positive urethral culture and/or the presence of specific IgM chlamydial antibody in serum at a titre of 1: ⩾2 as evidence of acute infection, 43% of patients were considered to have acute *C. trachomatis* infection, compared with 50% of men with NGU who were similarly studied. The spread of titres of IgG and IgM antibodies in random sera obtained during the period of active arthritis from patients with SARA and from appropriate control groups is shown in Fig. 11 a and b. It may be of some interest that the only spondylitic patient to have repeatedly high titres also had bilateral knee effusions. All patients with arthritis who had positive urethral cultures showed high titres of IgG serum antibody (Fig. 12), with a GMT of 188, compared with 15.2 amongst isolate-positive men with uncomplicated NGU. It was also possible to show in this study that eight patients studied serially who had evidence of chlamydial genital infection at the onset of joint disease had significant (four-fold or greater) rises and/or falls in IgG and IgM antibody titres during the course of their disease. The typical changes of a response to acute infection were seen in these patients (Fig. 13). In a recent study [103] of 31 patients (seven women) with probable reactive arthritis associated with sexually transmitted genital infection, 17 (59%) were found to have titres of serum IgG antibody of 1: ⩾64: this included all seven females.

    This exaggerated antibody response to *C. trachomatis* in acute SARA is significant in two respects. First, it provides powerful evidence of acute *C. trachomatis* infection at the time of onset arthritis. Second, it may provide a clue to important

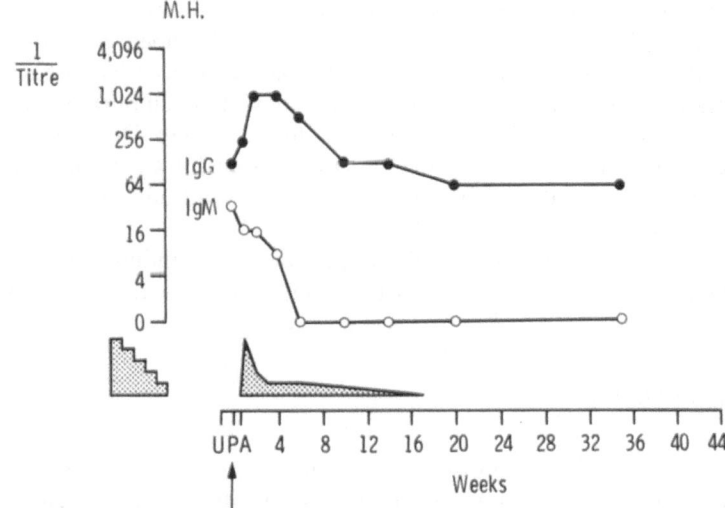

Fig. 13. Serial changes in titre of IgG and IgM chlamydial antibody during the course of SARA in one male patient. *U*, onset of urethritis symptoms; *A*, onset of arthritis symptoms; *P*, presentation to hospital. *Hatched area* indicates duration and severity of rheumatic symptoms

pathogenic mechanisms. It could reflect an especially large antigen load or an unusually effective mode of presentation of antigen to the immune system. Experience on both SARA and NGU [96] suggest that it is not due to an anamnestic reaction and that it does not solely reflect previous exposure to antigen. High antibody titres might result from reduction in normal suppressor cell activity, which might in turn be a direct effect of chlamydial infection, the result of pre-existing virus infection in immunocompetent cells or a genetically determined phenomenon. Since this phenomenon of high antibody production is indirectly linked with the presence of HLA-B27, both being found in individuals with reactive arthritis, it is possible that this reflects a specific genetic anomaly somewhere in the intricate chain of processes involved in antibody synthesis.

Cell-Mediated Immunity and Reiter's Syndrome

The assessment of cellular sensitization to chlamydial antigens has been hampered by the lack of ideal chlamydial antigen preparations. Several groups have used crude extracts of chlamydial elementary bodies (usually LGV strains or *C. psittaci*) in the lymphocyte transformation test. Two French groups [104, 105] have demonstrated increased cellular reactivity in 75% of patients with Reiter's syndrome. Similar results were obtained [104] amongst patients with uncomplicated chlamydial-inclusion-positive urethritis, though not in patients with inclusion-negative urethritis. Pattin and colleagues [105] also noted positive lymphocyte transformation tests in 50% of patients with spondylitis, irrespective of the presence of peripheral arthritis. They noted, in addition, a high proportion of positive tests amongst patients with Reiter's syndrome acquired in North Africa, probably of dysenteric origin, and in a more recent study Amor and colleagues [106] noted the presence of urethral chlamydial-like inclusion bodies, positive lymphocyte transformation tests to chlamydial antigen and raised titres of chlamydial serum antibody in two of six patients with Reiter's syndrome associated with diarrhoea. Subsequently, Martin and colleagues [106 a] have demonstrated clearly enhanced lymphocyte transformation responses in Reiter's syndrome compared with uncomplicated urethritis.

Skin testing has been used only to a limited extent: Dunlop and colleagues [107], using extracts of oculogenital and LGV strains of *C. trachomatis,* found positive skin tests in nine of 13 patients with Reiter's syndrome, as compared with nine of 50 men with uncomplicated NGU.

These data clearly strongly support the other findings of an enhanced state of antichlamydial immune reactivity in some patients with reactive arthritis.

Conclusion

The wealth of new information that has become available during last decade has caused considerable revision of our views on the concept of Reiter's syndrome. This has led to the formation of many critical questions, though has provided few of the answers so far. From a clinical viewpoint the concept of reactive arthritis is useful as, although the condition may be recognized by a more or less characteristic clinical picture, it is defined by the relationship between arthritis and infection, rather than by the presence of particular clinical features. Both clinically and for the purposes of research it is essential to separate the various aetiological groups of reactive arthritis, though it has to be recognized that this is not possible in all cases. The concept of reactive arthritis is based on the hypothesis that the joint lesions are sterile: data relating to this assumption are, however, conflicting and incomplete, so that this should be regarded as a working hypothesis only whilst further work is undertaken to establish or refute it.

Approximately one-half to two-thirds of patients with SARA have acute *C. trachomatis* genital infection at the time of onset of their arthritis. Furthermore, they have evidence of increased humoral and probably cellular reactivity to chlamydial antigens as compared with individuals with uncomplicated *C. trachomatis* genital infections, and this may be the basis of an important though currently somewhat enigmatic clue to the basic pathogenetic mechanisms. A substantial minority of patients with SARA and the majority of those with reactive arthritis of other causes do not have chlamydial infection. It has been suggested that infection by *Ureaplasma urealyticum, Neisseria gonorrhoeae* or herpes simplex might be important in some of these patients, though supporting evidence for such contentions is insubstantial.

It is likely that reactive arthritis is a genetically programmed "reaction pattern" which may be initiated by many different infectious agents, the patient's genetic "soil" being of far greater importance than the nefarious but non-specific seeds which set the process in motion.

References

1. Bywaters EGL (1968) The Cheshire Cat syndrome. Postgrad Med J 44: 19–22
2. Bauer W, Engleman EP (1942) Syndrome of unknown aetiology characterised by urethritis, conjunctivitis and arthritis (so-called Reiter's disease). Trans Assoc Am Physicians 57: 307–313
3. Hancock JAH (1964) Reiter's disease. In: King A (ed) Recent advances in venerology, 1st edn. Churchill, London, pp 398–471
4. Arnett FC, McClusky OE, Schachter BZ, Lordon RE (1976) Incomplete Reiter's syndrome: discriminating features and HL-AW27 in diagnosis. Ann Intern Med 84: 8–12
5. Reiter H (1916) Über eine bisher unerkannte Spirochaeteninfektion (spirochaetosis arthritica). Dtsch Med Wochenschr 42: 1535–1536
6. Aho K, Ahvonen P, Lassus A, Sievers K, Tiilikainen A (1974) HL-A27 in reactive arthritis. A study of *Yersinia* arthritis and Reiter's disease. Arthritis Rheum 17: 521–526
7. Dumonde DC, Steward MW (1978) The role of microbial infection in rheumatic disease. In: Scott JT (ed) Copeman's textbook of the rheumatic diseases, 5th edn. Churchill Livingstone, Edinburgh, pp 221–258
8. Wright V, Moll JMH (1976) The seronegative spondarthritides – a new concept in "seronegative polyarthritis". North-Holland, Amsterdam, pp 29–80
9. Rosenthal L, Olhagen B, Ek S (1980) Aseptic arthritis after gonorrhoea. Ann Rheum Dis 39: 141–146
10. Koteen H (1945) Lymphogranuloma venereum. Medicine (Baltimore) 24: 1–69
11. Sonck CE (1951) Erythema nodosum in connection with lymphogranuloma inguinale. Acta Derm Venerol (Stockh) 31: 517–567
12. Julkunen H, Pietila K (1964) Chronic salpingo-oophoritis and rheumatoid spondylitis. Acta Rheum Scand 10: 209–214
13. Szanto E, Hagenfeldt K (1979) Sacro-iliitis and salpingitis. Scand J Rheumatol 8: 129–135

14. Romanus R (1953) Pelvo-spondylitis ossificans in the male and genito-urinary infection. Acta Med Scand 145 [suppl. 280]: 172–178
15. Mason RM, Murray RS, Oates JK, Young AC (1958) Prostatitis and ankylosing spondylitis. Br Med J 1: 748–751
16. Kaslow RA, Ryder RW, Calin A (1979) A search for Reiter's syndrome after an outbreak of *Shigella sonnei* dysentery. J Rheumatol 6: 562–566
17. Gabrielle H, Hugonot G, Duval M (1938) Syndrome urétro-articulaire au cours d'une entérite à lamblia. Lyon-Med 162: 299–304
18. Graby M, Graby A (1949) Syndrome de Fiessinger-Leroy avec polyneurite. Can Med J 4: 93–96
19. Ravin JG (1972) Reiter's syndrome in childhood. A sequel to traveller's diarrhoea. J Ped Ophthalmol 9: 87–89
20. Shagrin JW, Frame B, Duncan H (1971) Polyarthritis in obese patients with intestinal bypass. Ann Intern Med 75: 377–380
21. Utsinger PD, Faber N, Shapiro RF (1978) Clinical and immunological study of the post-intestinal bypass arthritis-dermatitis snydrome. Arthritis Rheum 21: 599–603
22. Van Patter WN, Bargen A, Dockerty MB, Feldman WH, Mayo CW, Waugh JM (1954) Regional enteritis. Gastroenterology 26: 347–450
23. Wright V, Watkinson G (1966) Articular complications of ulcerative colitis. Am J Proctol 17: 107–115
24. Hawkins CF, Farr N, Morris CJ, Hoare AM, Williamson N (1976) Detection by electron microscopy of rod-shaped organisms in synovial membrane from a patient with the arthritis of Whipple's disease. Ann Rheum Dis 35: 502–509
25. Brewerton DA, Caffrey M, Hart FD, James DCO, Nicholls A, Sturrock RD (1973) Ankylosing spondylitis and HL-A27. Lancet 1: 904–907
26. Schlosstein L, Terasaki PI, Bluestone R, Pearson CM (1973) High association of the HL-A antigen W27 with ankylosing spondylitis. N Eng J Med 288: 704–706
27. Moll JMH, Haslock I, Macrae IF, Wright V (1974) Association between ankylosing spondylitis, psoriatic arthritis, Reiter's disease, the intestinal arthropathies and Behçet's syndrome. Medicine (Baltimore) 53: 343–364
28. Brewerton DA, Caffrey M, Nicholls A, Walters D, Oates JK, James DCO (1973) Reiter's disease and HL-A27. Lancet 2: 996–998
29. Woodrow JC, Treanor B, Usher N (1974) The HL-A system in Reiter's syndrome. Tissue Antigens 4: 533–540
30. Harris JRW, Gelsthorpe K, Doughty RW, Lee D, Morton RF (1975) HL-A27 and W10 in Reiter's syndrome and non-specific urethritis. Acta Derm Venereol (Stockh) 55: 127–130
31. Morris R, Metzger AL, Bluestone R, Terasaki PI (1974) HL-W27 – a clue to the diagnosis and pathogenesis of Reiter's syndrome. N Engl J Med 290: 554–556
32. Caughey DE, Douglas R, Wilson W, Hassall IB (1975) HLA antigens in Europeans and Maoris with rheumatic fever and rheumatic heart disease. J Rheumatol 2: 319–321
33. Friis J (1975) HL-A27 in *Neisseria*-infected patients with arthritis. Scand J Rheumatol 8 [suppl abstr 30]: 12
34. Robitaille A, Cockburn C, James DCO, Ansell BM (1976) HLA frequencies in less common arthropathies. Ann Rheum Dis 35: 271–273
35. Cleland LG, Hay JAR, Milazzo SC (1975) The relation of HL-A27 to disease pattern in seronegative rheumatoid arthritis. Scand J Rheumatol 8 [suppl abstr] 30: 20
36. Brewerton DA, Caffrey M, Nicholls A, Walters D, James DCO (1973) Acute anterior uveitis and HL-A27. Lancet 2: 994–996
37. Woodrow JC, Mapstone R, Anderson J, Usher N (1975) HL-A27 and anterior uveitis. Tissue Antigens 6: 116–120
38. Lawrence JS (1974) Family survey of Reiter's disease. Br J Vener Dis 50: 140–145
39. Woodrow JC (1977) Histocompatibility antigens and rheumatic diseases. Semin Arthritis Rheum 6: 257–276
40. Svejgaard A, Morling N, Platz P, Ryder LP, Thomsen N (1981) HLA and disease associations with special reference to mechanisms. Transplant Proc 13: 913–917
41. Keat A (1982) HLA-linked disease susceptibility and reactive arthritis. J Infect 5: 227–239

42. Keat AC (1983) Reiter's syndrome and reactive arthritis in perspective. N Engl J Med 309: 1606-1615
43. Yates DB, Maini RN, Scott JT, Sloper JC (1975) Complement activation in Reiter's syndrome. Ann Rheum Dis 34: 468 (abstract)
44. Baldassare AR, Weiss TD, Tsai CC, Arthur RE, Moore TL, Zuckner J (1981) Immunoprotein deposition in synovial tissue in Reiter's syndrome. Ann Rheum Dis 40: 281-285
45. Lovgren O (1956) Syndroma Reiter. Acta Rheum Scand 2: 11-16
46. Keat AC, Maini RN, Pegrum GD, Scott JT (1979) The clinical features and HLA-associations of reactive arthritis associated with non-gonococcal urethritis. Q J Med 48: 323-324
47. Leirisalo M, Skylv G, Kousa M, Voipio-Pulkki L-M, Suoranta H, Nissila M, Hvidman L, Damm Nielssen E, Svejgaard A, Tiilikainen A, Laitinen O (1982) Follow-up study on patients with Reiter's disease and reactive arthritis with special reference to HLA-B27. Arthritis Rheum 25: 249-259
48. Oates JK, Young AC (1959) Sacroiliitis in Reiter's disease. Br Med J 1: 1013-1015
49. Sholkoff SD, Glickman MG, Steinbach HL (1971) The radiographic pattern of polyarthritis in Reiter's syndrome. Arthritis Rheum 14: 551-555
50. Steinbach HL, Jensen PS (1976) Roentgenographic changes in the arthritides (part II). Semin Arthritis Rheum 5: 203-246
51. Russell AS, Lentle BC, Percy JS (1975) Investigation of sacroiliac disease: comparative evaluation of radiological and radionuclide techniques. J Rheumatol 2: 45-51
52. Szanto E, Lindvall N (1978) Quantitative ^{99m}Tc pertechnetate scanning. Scand J Rheumatol 7: 93-96
53. Russell AS, Davis P, Percy JS, Lentle BC (1977) The sacroiliitis of acute Reiter's syndrome. J Rheumatol 4: 293-296
54. Good AE (1965) Reiter's disease and ankylosing spondylitis. Acta Rheum Scand 11: 305-317
55. Granger RG, Nicol CS (1959) Pelvic infection as a cause of bilateral sacroiliac arthritis and ankylosing spondylitis. Br J Vener Dis 35: 92-98
56. Csonka GW (1959) Significance of sacroiliitis in Reiter's disease. Br J Vener Dis 35: 77-80
57. Sairanen E, Paronen I, Mahonen H (1969) Reiter's syndrome: a follow-up study. Acta Med Scand 185: 57-63
58. Paronen I (1948) Reiter's disease. A study of 344 cases observed in Finland. Acta Med Scand 131 [suppl 212]: 1-112
59. Calin A, Fries JF (1975) Striking prevalence of ankylosing spondylitis in "healthy" W-27 positive males and females. N Engl J Med 293: 835-839
60. Cohen LM, Mittal KK, Schmid FR (1976) Increased risk for spondylitis stigmata in apparently healthy HLA-W27 men. Ann Intern Med 84: 1-7
60a. Kidd KK, Bernoco D, Carbonara OA, Daneo V, Steiger U, Ceppellini R (1977) Genetic analysis of HLA-associated diseases. "The illness-susceptible" gene frequency and sex ratio in ankylosing spondylitis. In: Dausset J, Svejgaard A (eds) HLA and disease. Munksgaard, Copenhagen, pp 72-79
60b. Woodrow JC, Nichol FE, Whitehouse GH (1983) Genetic studies in ankylosing spondylitis. Br J Rheumatol [suppl] 22: 12-17
61. Keat AC, Barnes RMR (1976) HL-A27-associated arthritis. Rheumatol Rehabil 15: 87-91
62. Brewerton DA (1978) Inherited susceptibility to rheumatic disease. J R Soc Med 71: 331-338
63. Niepel GA, Kostka D, Kopecky S, Manca S (1966) Enthesopathy. Acta Rheum Balneol Pistiniana 1: 9-14
64. Mladenovic V, Kerimovic D, Keserovic P (1974) Enthesopathies in Reiter's disease. Acta Rheum Belgradiensa 4: 165-169
65. Thambar IV, Dunlop R, Thin RN, Huskisson EC (1977) Circinate vulvitis in Reiter's syndrome. Br J Vener Dis 53: 260-262
66. Auckland G (1951) Keratoderma blennorrhagica. Report of a case and suggestions concerning its nature. Br J Vener Dis 27: 143-149
67. Weinberger HW, Ropes MW, Kulka P, Bauer W (1962) Reiter's syndrome, clinical and pathological observations. Medicine (Baltimore) 41: 35-91
68. Kousa M (1978) Clinical observations on Reiter's disease with special reference to the venereal and non-venereal aetiology. Acta Derm Venereol (Stockh) 58 [suppl]: 1-81
69. Lassus A (1975) Circinate erosive balanitis. Ann Rheum Dis 34 [suppl]: 54

70. Ahvonen P (1972) Human yersiniosis in Finland. II Clinical features. Ann Clin Res 4: 39–48
71. Zewi M (1947) Morbus Reiteri. Acta Ophthalmol (Copenh) 25: 47–60
72. Mattsson R (1955) Recurrent retinitis in Reiter's disease. Acta Ophthalmol (Copenh) 33: 403–407
73. Baxter CR (1946) Reiter's disease. Br Med J 2: 858
74. Batchelor RCL (1946) Penicillin in treatment of venereal disease – year's experience in a civilian clinic. Edinb Med J 53: 31–36
75. Laitinen O, Leirisalo M, Allander E (1975) Rheumatic fever and *Yersinia* arthritis, criteria and diagnostic problems in a changing disease pattern. Scand J Rheumatol 4: 145–157
76. Hall WH, Feingold S (1953) A study of 23 cases of Reiter's syndrome. Ann Intern Med 38: 533–536
77. Masbernard A (1959) Le syndrome de Fiessinger-Leroy-Reiter, l'étude de 80 cas observés en Tunisie. Rev Rhum Mal Osteoartic 26: 21–26
78. Csonka GW, Oates JK (1967) Pericarditis and electrocardiographic changes in Reiter's syndrome. Br Med J 1: 866–869
79. Yates DB, Scott JT (1975) Cardiac valvular disease in chronic inflammatory disorders of connective tissue: factors influencing survival. Ann Rheum Dis 34: 321–325
80. Csonka GW (1958) Involvement of the nervous system in Reiter's syndrome. Ann Rheum Dis 17: 334–336
81. Oates JK, Hancock JAH (1959) Neurological symptoms and lesions occurring in the course of Reiter's disease. Amer J Med Sci 238: 79–83
82. Lindsay-Rea R (1947) Un cas de maladie de Reiter. Trans Ophthalmol Soc UK 67: 241–242
83. Caughey DE, Wakem CG (1973) A fatal case of Reiter's disease complicated by amyloidosis. Arthritis Rheum 16: 695–700
84. Csonka GW (1958) The course of Reiter's syndrome. Br Med J 1: 1088–1090
85. Fox R, Calin A, Gerber RC, Gibson D (1979) The chronicity of symptoms and disability in Reiter's syndrome. An analysis of 131 consecutive patients. Ann Intern Med 91: 190–193
86. McClusky OE, Lorden RE, Arnett FC (1974) HL-A27 in Reiter's syndrome and psoriatic arthritis – a genetic factor in disease susceptibility and expression. J Rheumatol 1: 263–268
87. Doury P, Pattin S, Roue R, Hainault J (1976) Relation entre antigène HLA-B27 et prognostic court terme du syndrome Fiessinger-Leroy-Reiter. Nouv Presse Méd 5: 2635
88. Laitinen O, Leirisalo M, Skylv G (1977) Relation between HLA-B27 and clinical features in patients with *Yersinia* arthritis. Arthritis Rheum 20: 11–21
89. Lindner K (1910) Zur Aetiologie Gonokokkenfreier Urethritis. Wien Klin Wochenschr 23: 283–284
90. Mendlowski B, Segre D (1960) Polyarthritis in sheep. I. Description of the disease and experimental transmission. Am J Vet Res 21: 68–73
91. Storz J (1961) Psittacosis agents as a cause of polyarthritis in cattle and sheep. Vet Med Rev 2/3: 125–139
92. Norton W (1969) Chlamydial infection in Reiter's syndrome. Annu Rev Med 20: 351–356
93. Smith DE, James PG, Schachter J, Engleman EP, Meyer KF (1973) Experimental bedsonial arthritis. Arthritis Rheum 16: 21–29
94. Siboulet A, Galestin P (1962) Arguments in favour of a virus aetiology of non-gonococcal urethritis illustrated by 3 cases of Reiter's disease. Br J Vener Dis 38: 209–211
95. Kousa M, Saikku P, Richmond S, Lassus A (1978) Frequent association of chlamydial infection with Reiter's syndrome. Sex Transm Dis 5: 57–61
96. Keat AC, Thomas BJ, Taylor-Robinson D, Pegrum GD, Maini RN, Scott JT (1980) Evidence of *Chlamydia trachomatis* infection in sexually acquired reactive arthritis. Ann Rheum Dis 39: 431–437
97. Jones BR, Al-Hussaini MK, Dunlop EMC (1964) Genital infection in association with TRIC virus infection of the eye. I. Isolation of virus from the urethra, cervix and eye: preliminary report. Br J Vener Dis 40: 19–24
98. Dawson CR, Schachter J, Ostler HE, Gilbert RN, Smith DE, Engleman EP (1970) Inclusion conjunctivitis and Reiter's disease in a married couple. Arch Ophthalmol 83: 300–306
99. Wang SP, Grayston JT (1970) Immunologic relationship between genital TRIC, lymphogranuloma venereum and related organisms in a new microtiter immunofluorescence test. Am J Ophthalmol 70: 367–375

100. Schachter J, Barnes MG, Jones JT, Engleman EP, Meyer KF (1966) Isolation of Bedsoniae from joints of patients with Reiter's syndrome. Proc Soc Exp Biol Med 122: 283-285
101. Kinsella TD, Norton WL, Ziff N (1968) Complement-fixing antibodies to bedsonian organisms in Reiter's syndrome and ankylosing spondylitis. Ann Rheum Dis 27: 241-244
102. Darougar S (1976) Immunology of *Chlamydia*. In: Catterall RD, Nicol CS (eds) Sexually transmitted diseases. Academic, New York, pp 111-120
103. Vilppula AH, Yli-kerttula UI, Ahlroos AK, Terho PE (1981) Chlamydial isolations and serology in Reiter's syndrome. Scand J Rheumatol 10: 181-185
104. Amor B, Kahan A, Lecoq F, Delbarre F (1972) Le test de transformation lymphoblastique par des antigènes bedsoniens (TTL Bedsonien). Rev Rhum 39: 671-676
105. Pattin S, Duørosoir J-L, Thabaut A, Doury P (1976) Le test de transformation lymphoblastique avec l'antigène bedsonien dans les syndromes de Fiessinger-Leroy-Reiter anciens, recentes et dans le spondylarthrite ankylosante. Rev Rhum 40: 643-649
106. Amor B, Kahan A, Orfila J, Thomas D (1979) Immunological evidence of chlamydial infection in Reiter's syndrome. Ann Rheum Dis 38: 116-118
106a. Martin DH, Pollock S, Kuo C-C, Wang S-P, Brunham KC, Holmes KK (1984) *C. trachomatis* infections in men with Reiter's syndrome. Ann Intern Med 100: 207-213
107. Dunlop EMC (1975) Non-specific genital infection. Laboratory aspects. In: Morton RS, Harris JR (eds) Recent advances in sexually transmitted diseases. Churchill Livingstone, Edinburgh, pp 267-295
108. Schachter J (1976) Can chlamydiae cause rheumatic disease? In: Dumonde DC (ed) Infection and immunology in the rheumatic diseases. Blackwell Scientific, Oxford, pp 151-157
109. Delbarre F, Amor B (1976) Ankylosing spondylitis and Reiter's syndrome: genetic and microbiological studies. In: Dumonde DC (ed) Infection and immunology in the rheumatic diseases. Blackwell Scientific, Oxford, pp 159-163
110. Dunlop EMC, Harper IA, Jones BR (1968) Seronegative polyarthritis. The Bedsoniae *(Chlamydia)* group of agents in Reiter's diseases. Ann Rheum Dis 27: 234-240
111. Ford DK (1968) Non-gonococcal urethritis and Reiter's syndrome: personal experience with aetiological studies during 15 years. Can Med Assoc J 99: 900-910
112. Ford DK, McCandlish L (1971) Isolation of human genital TRIC agents in non-gonococcal urethritis and Reiter's disease. Br J Vener Dis 47: 196-197
113. Vaughan-Jackson JD, Dunlop EMC, Darougar S, Dwyer R, Jones BR (1972) Chlamydial infection. Results of tests for *Chlamydia* in patients suffering from acute Reiter's disease compared with results of tests from the genital tract and rectum in patients with ocular infection due to TRIC agents. Br J Vener Dis 48: 445-451
114. Gordon FB, Quan AL, Steinman TI, Phillip RN (1973) Chlamydial isolates from Reiter's syndrome. Br J Vener Dis 49: 376-380
115. Shatkin AA, Popov VL, Scherbakova NI (1976) Morphology of Halprowia *(Chlamydia)* isolated in Reiter's syndrome. J Microbiol Epidemiol Immunobiol 4: 60-64
116. Harisijades S, Mladenovic V, Markovic L, Kerimovic D, Nedeljkovic M (1975) Uloga *Hlamidija* u etiologiji Reiterove bolesti. Rcumatizam (Zagreb) 22: 85-89

Subject Index